Alcohol in America
Taking Action to Prevent Abuse

Steve Olson in collaboration with Dean R. Gerstein

Foreword by Elizabeth Hanford Dole

Panel on Alternative Policies Affecting the Prevention
of Alcohol Abuse and Alcoholism
Commission on Behavioral and Social Sciences and Education
National Research Council

567157

NATIONAL ACADEMY PRESS
Washington, D.C.   1985

National Academy Press   2101 Constitution Avenue, NW   Washington, DC 20418

This publication is based on two reports from the Commission on Behavioral and Social Sciences and Education of the National Research Council: *Alcohol and Public Policy: Beyond the Shadow of Prohibition* (Washington, D.C.: National Academy Press, 1981) and *Toward the Prevention of Alcohol Problems: Government, Business, and Community Action* (Washington, D.C.: National Academy Press, 1984). It has been reviewed according to procedures approved by a Report Review Committee consisting of members of the National Academy of Sciences, the National Academy of Engineering, and the Institute of Medicine.

The National Research Council was established by the National Academy of Sciences in 1916 to associate the broad community of science and technology with the Academy's purposes of furthering knowledge and of advising the federal government. The Council operates in accordance with general policies determined by the Academy under the authority of its congressional charter of 1863, which establishes the Academy as a private, nonprofit, self-governing membership corporation. The Council has become the principal operating agency of both the National Academy of Sciences and the National Academy of Engineering in the conduct of their services to the government, the public, and the scientific and engineering communities. It is administered jointly by both Academies and the Institute of Medicine. The National Academy of Engineering and the Institute of Medicine were established in 1964 and 1970, respectively, under the charter of the National Academy of Sciences.

Library of Congress Cataloging-in-Publication Data

Olson, Steve, 1956-
    Alcohol in America.

    Bibliography: p.
    1. Alcoholism—United States—Prevention.
    2. Drinking of alcoholic beverages—United States.
    II. Gerstein, Dean R.   II. National Research Council (U.S.). Panel on
Alternative Policies Affecting the Prevention of Alcohol Abuse and
Alcoholism.   III. Title.
HV5296.063 1985   362.2'9286   85-13667
ISBN 0-309-03449-3

Printed in the United States of America

Foreword

THIS BOOK IS A THOUGHTFUL and useful contribution to the worthiest of national causes: continuing public awareness of alcohol abuse.

When I became Secretary of Transportation, I resolved to have no higher priority than safety—on our highways, railways, airways, and waterways. I learned very quickly that alcohol abuse is a major cause of many transportation accidents, whether it is a drunk driver on our highways or a recreational boater who has had one drink too many. Alcohol abuse affects transportation safety in a very dramatic and tragic way. More than 44,000 people were killed on our highways last year, many of them by drunk drivers. Thousands of others were maimed and injured, and millions of dollars of property were destroyed. The tragedy does not end with the victims. The injury and heartache of families and loved ones linger.

Our campaign to get drunk drivers off our highways aroused public consciousness throughout America, and the public outcry to stop senseless killing on our highways is just beginning to pay dividends in lives saved and accidents prevented. The campaign against drunk drivers is strong today because of a grassroots movement that began at the local level, in the clubs, the churches, the city halls, courthouses, and state houses all across America. As a result we have stronger laws against drunk drivers and stricter enforcement. We must keep this momentum going. We need to work for continuing awareness of all the many problems associated with alcohol abuse.

This book is a useful tool for maintaining that heightened awareness. It deserves to be read by parents, teachers, students, legislators, community organizers, government officials, and anyone searching for ways to translate concern about alcohol abuse into action aimed at preventing it.

I congratulate the National Academy of Sciences on giving us this book, which provides just the kind of timely, provocative, and practical contribution that the research community can make toward action on one of our most pressing national concerns. I urge you to take this book home, take it to your hearts, and, where it strikes a responsive chord, take action.

ELIZABETH HANFORD DOLE, *Secretary*
U.S. Department of Transportation

August 1985

Preface

*I*N 1978 THE NATIONAL RESEARCH COUNCIL initiated a study of alternative policies affecting the prevention of alcohol abuse and alcoholism. The study panel brought together researchers in anthropology, economics, education, epidemiology, psychiatry, psychology, and sociology along with experts on the analysis of historical, legal, and political dimensions of public policy. A list of its members appears on page 119.

In 1981 the panel issued a report entitled *Alcohol and Public Policy: Beyond the Shadow of Prohibition*, which thoroughly reviewed the relevant research literature and policy questions, and concluded:

- Alcohol problems are permanent, because drinking is an important and ineradicable part of this society and culture.
- Alcohol problems tend to be so broadly felt and distributed as to be a general social problem, even though they are excessively prevalent in a relatively small fraction of the population.
- The possibilities for reducing the problem by preventive measures are modest but real and should increase with experience; they should not be ignored because of ghosts from the past.

Shortly after this report was published, the National Institute on Alcohol Abuse and Alcoholism (the federal agency that had commissioned the study) asked that the National Research Council organize a conference for some of the report's authors, other researchers, and participants from all walks of life concerned with alcohol-related problems to examine the study panel's findings and discuss their implications for public policy and private action. The conference papers and discussions were turned into a book, *Toward the Prevention of Alcohol Problems: Government, Business, and Community Action*, published in 1984.

The present volume represents a third phase of this National Research Council effort to inform and advance the discussion of preventive approaches to alcohol problems. Steve Olson was commissioned by the National Academy Press, publisher of the two earlier volumes, to distill those works into a shorter and more accessible form, with advice from members of the study panels responsible for those efforts, other reviewers, and me. The present volume, while derived from the earlier efforts, has been written and reviewed with an eye toward current trends in research on prevention and relevant areas of public and private action. A list of further readings and resources appears as an appendix.

The subject of preventing alcohol problems is itself representative of a broad range of public concerns that have substantial, though not always well-known, technical and scientific dimensions. This type of extension and guide to more technical National Research Council activities and reports is a relatively new enterprise. It symbolizes a commitment by the National Research Council, the National Academy Press, and their parent organizations, the National Academy of Sciences, the National Academy of Engineering, and the Institute of Medicine, to place greater emphasis on the provision of advice and information not only to the federal government but also to other levels of government and to the public.

DEAN R. GERSTEIN, *Study Director*
Panel on Alternative Policies
Affecting the Prevention of
Alcohol Abuse and Alcoholism

Contents

Foreword
Elizabeth Hanford Dole iii

1. Drinking in America 1

2. Why Prevention? 20

3. Preventing Drunk Driving 32

4. The Price and Availability of Alcohol 45

5. What Servers Can Do 62

6. Drinking by Young People 70

7. Drinking and the Mass Media 82

8. Reducing Environmental Risk 95

9. Summary and Outlook 104

Guide to Information Sources 113

Panel Members 119

Index 121

Alcohol in America
Taking Action to Prevent Abuse

1

Drinking in America

A PARENT RAISES A GLASS of champagne to toast a newly
wedded couple. Friends gather after work or on weekends to talk, drink, and relax. A host produces a prized
liqueur to top off a special meal. These are some of the images
that come to mind when one thinks about drinking in America.

There are other, darker images of drinking: an intoxicated
driver losing control of a car; a family argument, fueled by
alcohol, escalating into a bloody assault; an employee missing
work due to increasingly frequent hangovers; a homeless man
clutching a bottle on a downtown street.

These images capture only part of what alcohol means in
America. But they are enough to demonstrate an important
point: drinking is a pervasive and deep-rooted feature of American life. Alcoholic beverages have been widely consumed
throughout American history, despite attempts by the government and other institutions to shape or even eliminate drinking
(see Figure 1-1).

The most radical attempt by the government to influence
drinking in the United States came in the years 1920 to 1933,
when the 18th Amendment to the U.S. Constitution brought
about Prohibition by banning the manufacture and sale of alcoholic beverages. Although majorities voted for Prohibition,
many people were opposed or indifferent to its enforcement,

1

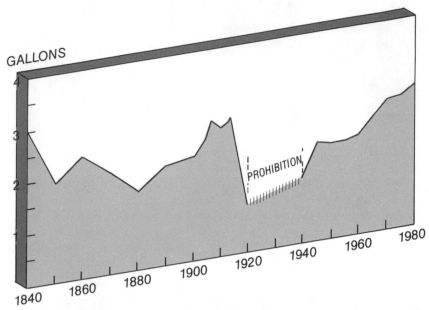

PER CAPITA CONSUMPTION OF ALCOHOL

FIGURE 1.1   The per capita consumption of alcoholic beverages in the United States has varied widely over the last 140 years. Before 1850, per capita consumption was falling from the high levels (6 to 7 gallons annually of pure alcohol per adult) characteristic of early America. Between 1850 and the beginning of World War I, it varied between 1.75 and 2.75 gallons, reaching its high point just before the war. Prohibition reduced per capita consumption to its lowest level in U.S. history, probably less than 1.5 gallons. Since about 1960, per capita consumption has again been rising, with a particularly marked acceleration in the 1960s. Today it is about what it was at the beginning of World War I. Source: Rutgers University Center of Alcohol Studies.

and the years of the "noble experiment" were a time of widespread and flagrant abuses of the law. But after its repeal by the 21st Amendment, Prohibition came to have a much broader meaning in the public consciousness. For many people it became an example of the futility of governmental attempts to legislate morality. The corollary of this view is that *any* attempt by the government to change drinking practices is doomed to fail.

The evidence does not support such a far-reaching conclusion. Prohibition demonstrated beyond doubt that drinking and the problems caused by drinking cannot simply be eliminated from the United States. But though such problems may always exist, their extent can grow smaller or larger depending on the steps taken—or not taken—to control them.

Drinking practices can change for an endless variety of reasons. Sometimes these changes are the result of small-scale, personal initiatives, such as an employer's threats or complaints, a spouse's encouragement, or the closing of a neighborhood bar. At other times these changes may come about through broader, public actions, such as mass media campaigns about drunk driving, changes in the laws governing when taverns may stay open, or shifts in the price of alcohol.

This book explores some of the private and public initiatives that can help reduce the substantial number of problems caused by drinking in the United States. Specifically, it focuses on those initiatives that can help *prevent* these problems before they occur or appear to be inevitable. Many of these prevention alternatives have been overlooked or slighted in the past. But they have the potential to make a major contribution. They can help produce, in the words of Mark Moore of Harvard University, a society "with fewer drinking problems—not zero drinking, not unlimited drinking, but some level of drinking with a much lower profile of harmful consequences than we now experience."

To lay the foundation for an examination of prevention policies, this chapter presents a brief history of drinking in America and explores the dimensions of drinking today. It asks the questions, how much do people drink and what are the consequences of that drinking? The second chapter introduces the general concept of prevention, distinguishing it from other approaches to alcohol problems, and examines some of the arguments for and against a prevention approach. The third chapter discusses perhaps the most visible challenge facing prevention today: drunk driving. Expanding on this focus, each succeeding chapter considers a different aspect of prevention, from the taxation of alcohol to educational campaigns to changes in the physical environment. The first part of the final chapter reviews the major conclusions of the book—and can be read as a summary of its findings—while the last part of the chapter looks toward the future of drinking and drinking problems in America.

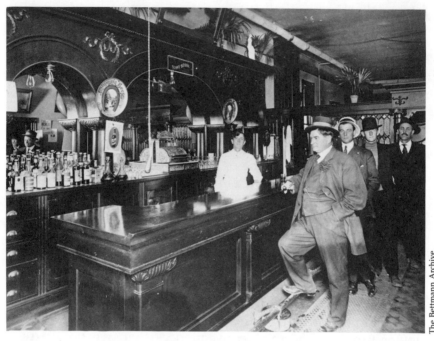

Drinking has been an integral part of American society throughout the country's history.

The Colonial and Temperance Views of Drinking

During the 150 years before the American Revolution the colonists of North America tended to regard heavy drinking as normal. According to Paul Aaron of Brandeis University and David Musto of Yale University, who review the historical research on drinking in America in *Alcohol and Public Policy: Beyond the Shadow of Prohibition,* "The colonists brought with them from Europe a high regard for alcoholic beverages. Distilled and fermented liquors were considered important and invigorating foods, whose restorative powers were a natural blessing. People in all regions and of all classes drank heavily. Wine and sugar were consumed at breakfast; at 11:00 and 4:00 workers broke for their 'bitters'; cider and beer were drunk at lunch and toddies for supper and during the evening." Alcohol was also a prominent feature of the colonists' social life. Such gatherings as barn raisings, fairs, and the mustering of militia were all accompanied by alcohol. In addition, taxes on alcohol were an important source of revenue for the fledgling colonial governments.

In this society drunkenness was seen as a personal failing, as a sin against a natural order. "Drunkenness was condemned and punished, but only as an abuse of a God-given gift," write Aaron and Musto. "Drink itself was not looked upon as culpable, any more than food deserved the blame for the sin of gluttony. Excess was personal indiscretion." The blame for drunkenness fell squarely on the shoulders of the drinker, not on rum or cider. Thus the solution to drunkenness was to chastise the moral character of the drunkard, whether in the stocks or from the pulpit.

During the 150 years after the revolution, a quite different view of drinking took hold. Many people came to see alcohol as an addicting and even poisonous drug. In this view, the drunkard was not a moral weakling but the victim of an alien substance. Alcohol could make normal people violent, dissolute, or degenerate. In this, it led to the breakdown of the family, which in turn weakened the social order. Moreover, because of alcohol's addictive qualities, even occasional drinkers flirted with danger at the rim of every cup.

This view found its institutional voice in the temperance societies of the 1800s and early 1900s. The mainly middle-class members of these societies renounced indulgence in liquor and other vices, often with evangelical fervor. In the 1830s these societies grew so rapidly that they prompted Alexis de Tocqueville's observation that America was a nation of joiners. By 1835, note Aaron and Musto, 1.5 million of America's 13 million citizens "had vowed never to consume ardent spirits again."

Though originally focused on self-improvement and exhortation, some of these groups developed political aims and fought for legislation at federal, state, and local levels to stem the ravages of alcohol. Several waves of prohibitionist sentiment swept the country in the nineteenth and early twentieth centuries, culminating in a surge of political action in the first two decades of this century. By 1916, 23 states had passed (mainly by referendum) prohibitionist laws of various kinds. Finally in 1920, after years of skilled single-issue politicking led by the Anti-Saloon League, the 18th Amendment extended prohibition to the nation as a whole.

Prohibition and the Alcoholism Movement

The 18th Amendment, drafted by the Anti-Saloon League in 1917 and ratified by the states in 1919, reads: "After one year from the ratification of this article the manufacture, sale, or transportation of intoxicating liquors within, the importation thereof into, or the exportation thereof from the United States and all territory subject to the jurisdiction thereof for beverage purposes is hereby prohibited." Close inspection of this wording reveals an interesting point. The amendment prohibits only the manufacture, sale, and transportation of intoxicating beverages, not their possession, consumption, or home production. This division was a foreshadowing of the difficulties to come. According to Aaron and Musto, "The 18th Amendment . . . was so full of compromise and disparity as to be 'amphibious' rather than 'dry.' "

The Anti-Saloon League and other temperance societies had a specific reason for trying to ban only the commerce of alcoholic beverages. They felt that once saloons and other drinking haunts were swept away, the taste for liquor would gradually die out. "According to Prohibitionist doctrine," write Aaron and Musto, "Americans had once been pure. A nefarious trade had robbed people of their reason and corrupted domestic and social integrity. The 18th Amendment represented a millennial triumph inaugurating personal self-restraint and national solidarity."

Nevertheless, even the temperance societies realized that this transformation would not occur overnight. The amendment gave people a year to dispose of their existing stocks, and the

Anti-Saloon League helped Congress write legislation to enforce the amendment. Thus was born the Volstead Act, a complicated and often ambiguous legal code. With 72 separate sections, the Volstead Act was an attempt to synthesize the best features of various state prohibitionist laws, but its contradictions and modifications of normal criminal procedures created enormous administrative and legal problems.

Furthermore, governments did not give a high priority to enforcing Prohibition. The Harding, Coolidge, and Hoover administrations committed a bare minimum of funds to enforcement; partly as a result, the Volstead Act was widely violated. Some of America's most notorious criminals date from this period. Bootlegging, moonshining, and speakeasies all thrived during Prohibition. Illegal marketeers developed a strong black market in booze, especially with drinkers willing to pay three to four times the prewar prices for it.

Illegal alcohol came from many sources. Among the largest, note Aaron and Musto, was alcohol used legally in industry. The 1920s were boom years for the young automotive industry, and because many of the new cars were enclosed they could be used in the winter. Their radiators therefore needed alcohol to use as antifreeze, and a portion of this increased alcohol production could be skimmed off and diverted to bootleggers.

People also made much more beer and wine at home. "During the first five years of Prohibition, the acreage of vineyards increased 700 percent," write Aaron and Musto. "The grapes were marketed as concentrate in 'blocks of port,' 'blocks of Rhine Wine,' and so forth and came with a warning: 'After dissolving the brick in a gallon of water, do not place the liquid in the jug away in the cupboard for 20 days, because then it would turn to wine.' "

Despite the flagrant abuses of Prohibition, much of the public remained strongly in favor of it. The elections of 1928 returned heavy majorities supporting the 18th Amendment to Congress. But the economic collapse that began the following year changed the situation drastically. The bulwarks of Prohibition crumbled in the face of a disaster that so clearly overshadowed alcohol as a source of social disorder and personal misery. The people who were fighting to repeal Prohibition gained a new argument. Relegalizing alcoholic beverages would both generate tax revenues and put Americans back to work. Roosevelt campaigned hard on these issues in his bid for the presidency. After his election in 1932, he promoted repeal as a key part of a recovery program, and in December 1933 the 21st Amendment ended what Roosevelt called the "damnable affliction of Prohibition."

Since the repeal of Prohibition, a view of drinking different from either the colonial or temperance views has steadily gained adherents. This view holds that excessive drinking is a chronic disease, a disease known as alcoholism. Neither the drinker nor the drink is morally evil. Rather the problem stems from a particular kind of chemistry between alcohol and certain drinkers. According to the alcoholism perspective, most people can drink with virtually no risk. But a minority—fine people in all other respects—cannot drink without succumbing to the disease. The only known cure for the disease is total abstinence. Thus it is the responsibility of the alcoholic or those who care about him or her to see that the disease is treated and abstinence is maintained.

No single view of alcohol completely shapes personal attitudes and public policies in the United States. Earlier views remain strong in certain ways, and alcohol policy in the years after Repeal was heavily shaped by the alcoholic beverage control movement, which held that the government should shape the context in which drinking took place to minimize its harmful consequences. But the alcoholism perspective lies at the heart of such organizations as Alcoholics Anonymous, and it provides the basis for many of the treatment programs that have arisen under medical auspices.

In recent years, the alcoholism concept has also found expression at the governmental level. The main federal agency concerned with alcohol problems is the National Institute on Alcohol Abuse and Alcoholism (NIAAA), which was formed in 1971 as part of the Alcohol, Drug Abuse, and Mental Health Administration. The NIAAA sponsors research on alcohol abuse and alcoholism (including the reports on which this book is based).

Also, many state and local treatment programs are based on the idea of alcoholism as a disease.

Compared with the temperance view, the alcoholism perspective is relatively new. But in the last 15 years it has shown itself capable of building a powerful institutional base. Like the temperance societies, the alcoholism movement has struck a chord among people who feel that their drinking or the drinking of people close to them threatens to overwhelm the rest of their lives. Also, the alcoholism movement, unlike the temperance movement, has been able to garner support from the alcoholic beverage industry. In terms of public attitudes and institutional backing, this conception promises to remain strong.

The Dimensions of Drinking

Alcoholic beverages are complex substances. Part drink, part food, and part drug, alcoholic beverages are consumed for reasons as diverse as thirst, culinary custom, and addiction. Alcohol is itself a source of calories, and most alcoholic beverages contain traces of other nutrients. Alcoholic beverages also rarely spoil and are free of most waterborne diseases. This was one reason why colonial Americans preferred alcohol to water, which was often considered impure and dangerous to drink.

Alcohol is also an intoxicating drug that can induce physical addiction. Depending on many different factors, it can stimulate or depress, make a person euphoric or sleepy, and heighten or reduce anxiety. The immediate effects of drinking vary widely in their degree and desirability, as evidenced by a rich vocabulary of descriptive terms. A person can be mellow, tipsy, or tight; plastered, soused, or loaded; dead drunk, under the table, or out cold.

The term *alcoholism* implies, at minimum, a loss of control over the intake of alcohol or an inability to stop drinking. Definitions and diagnostic criteria vary beyond this core element, but they generally refer to the quantities of alcohol consumed, the recurrence of physical signs such as blackouts, habits such as morning drinking or binge drinking, disruption of life such as job absenteeism or arrest, and tolerance or withdrawal symptoms.[1] Alcoholism is a subset of the broader category of *excessive drinking*, *alcohol abuse*, or *problem drinking*, terms which are used in this book to characterize all problems caused by or associated with drinking. In this broader category, the amount consumed may be considered excessive, even though it is not repeated on a regular basis.

The measurement of consumption generally begins with the amount of alcohol in a drink. The common denominator joining the three types of alcoholic beverages—beer, wine, and distilled spirits—is ethyl alcohol, which is present in quite different concentrations in each type of beverage. Beer is generally 3 to 6 percent alcohol by volume, with "light" beer at the low end and "malt liquor" at the high end; wine is generally 10 to 20 percent alcohol, with table wine low and fortified "dessert" wine high; and spirits are today generally bottled at 40 percent alcohol (80 proof), with higher proofs for special labels.

The way that beverages are ordinarily served in individual drinks greatly reduces these disparities in alcohol concentration. A 12-ounce can of 4 percent beer, a 4-ounce serving of 12 percent wine, and a cocktail with 1.2 ounces of 80-proof spirits contain identical amounts of alcohol. Obviously, commercial vendors and private hosts can freely vary the size and dilution of their drinks. But as an overall rule of thumb, a single drink typically contains in the neighborhood of one-half fluid ounce of pure alcohol, about 12 grams by weight.

Once consumed and passed from the stomach to the small intestine, alcohol is rapidly absorbed and diffused throughout

---

[1] For more detailed definitions, see *Diagnostic and Statistical Manual of Mental Disorders*, 3rd Edition, Washington, D.C.: American Psychiatric Association, 1980; Lester Grinspoon, ed., "Part IV: Alcohol Abuse and Dependence," pp. 299-389 in *Psychiatry Update, The American Psychiatric Association Annual Review*, Volume III, Washington, D.C.: American Psychiatric Press, 1984; Jeffrey H. Boyd, Myrna M. Weissman, W. Douglas Thompson, and Jerome K. Myers, Different definitions of alcoholism, I: Impact of seven definitions on prevalence rates in a community survey, *American Journal of Psychiatry* 140(1983):1309-1313; and Division of Health Promotion and Disease Prevention, Institute of Medicine, *Alcoholism, Alcohol Abuse and Related Problems: Opportunities for Research*, Washington, D.C.: National Academy of Sciences, 1980.

the body. The most common laboratory measure of intoxication is blood alcohol concentration, or BAC. This measurement is typically expressed in terms of the weight of alcohol that is found in a standard volume of blood, also known as the "grams percent" figure. Thus a reading of .10 percent BAC means that there are .10 grams of pure alcohol per 100 milliliters of blood.

The liver metabolizes alcohol at an average rate of about one drink per hour, so that any drinking in excess of this rate will elevate the BAC. However, this clearance rate and other physiological characteristics vary greatly, making some people more sensitive to alcohol than others. Also, an individual's responses can differ as a result of aging, illness, fatigue, or tolerance. Body weight, gender, the spacing of drinks, metabolic rates, how much food has been eaten, the drinker's expectations, and even the expectations of others influence the degree of intoxication. A skinny teenager anticipating a big night with friends can become exhilarated on a quantity of alcohol that would produce virtually no effect in a heavy middle-aged man who had just finished a large dinner.

The BAC correlates reliably with loss of coordination, especially for such tasks as precise reasoning, eye-hand coordination, and balance while moving. Intoxication also makes people generally less alert in scanning the environment for hazards, less reliable in interpreting what is observed, and inclined to relax or be easily distracted. At a BAC of 0.05 percent, which for most people requires three or more drinks within an hour, physical skills begin to deteriorate. At BACs of 0.08 to 0.10 percent, most jurisdictions consider a person legally intoxicated. At BACs of 0.15 to 0.30 percent a person can grow stuporous or lose consciousness. Above 0.30 percent a person can die due to respiratory depression or inhaling vomit while unconscious.

Another important measure of drinking, besides the amount consumed in a single drinking episode, is the average amount of alcohol drunk over many drinking episodes. There are several ways to obtain such statistics, but the most valuable source of information is household surveys of the general population. These surveys do have limitations, however. Most important, people report drinking only about two-thirds of the total amount of alcohol purchased. Nevertheless, because relatively small changes in the overall figures can account for the alcohol that goes unreported, such surveys provide a fairly good idea of how drinking habits are distributed across the population.

The most remarkable result of these surveys is how much of the adult population does not drink or drinks very little (see Figure 1-2). Approximately one third of all adults report not having drunk any alcohol over the previous year. This figure is down from the late 1950s, when 45 percent of all adults reported abstaining. But it remains higher than in Canada or any of the countries of western Europe. For the nation as a

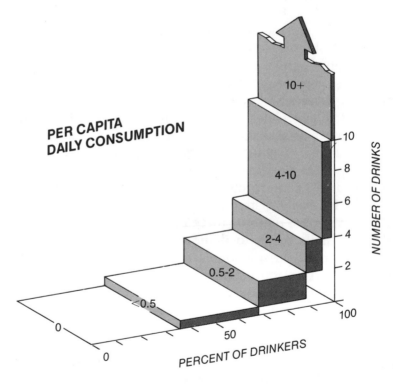

FIGURE 1.2 Surveys of the general population indicate that roughly a third of the adult population in the United Stated does not drink, while another third has an average of less than three drinks per week. Such surveys account for only about two thirds of the total amount of alcohol purchased, but they give a fairly good idea of how consumption is distributed across the population. Source: Rand Corporation (Santa Monica, California).

whole, about 27 percent of men don't drink, compared with 42 percent of women. This widespread abstinence testifies to the continued strength of the temperance outlook in America.

Another third of the adult population reports drinking very little—fewer than three drinks per week. Thus two thirds of the adult population is very temperate. The next fifth or so of the population averages about two drinks per day. About the next tenth of all adults average three or more drinks per day. Twice as many men as women report this level of consumption. Finally, the last 1 to 4 percent of the population averages 10 or more drinks per day. Almost all people being treated for alcoholism report drinking this much, although this level of consumption is not a hard and fast definition of the disorder.

Another standard way to assess the average consumption of alcohol in a given area is to divide the total amount of alcohol sold in that area by the area's adult population. The resulting per capita consumption rate can be skewed by large numbers of tourists, by the importation or exportation of alcohol (border-crossing "liquor runs," for example), and by unreported production (including production at home). But over a large area, such as an entire country, per capita consumption can be estimated fairly well.

The per capita consumption of pure alcohol in the United States is about two and three-quarter gallons per year, which corresponds to just under an ounce a day, or close to two drinks. Of course, this overall figure disguises a wide variation in the drinking habits of individuals. The per capita consumption rate actually depends strongly on the drinking patterns of a minority of the population. A third of the adult population drinks 95 percent of all the alcohol consumed, with 5 percent of the population accounting for half of the overall total. Thus, changes in consumption among a small fraction of the population have a large impact on per capita consumption.

The Consequences of Drinking

Given the prevalence and variety of drinking in America, it is not surprising that the link between drinking and the consequences of drinking is very complex. Drinking never occurs in a social or psychological vacuum. It is done at a certain time, in a certain place, often in the company of others, and in the context of profoundly intricate personal and social histories. All of these factors can influence what the consequences of drinking, whether positive or negative, will be.

One way to begin untangling the links between the use of alcohol and its consequences is through an analysis of drinking practices. These practices have two components: the amount and distribution of alcohol consumed, and the settings and activities associated with drinking. Either of these aspects can play a critical role in determining the consequences of drinking. For instance, the more often a person is drunk, the greater the chance of being drunk in the wrong place at the wrong time. The frequency of drunkenness may also signal the onset of unreliability in a spouse or employee.

The setting in which a person drinks can also be a pivotal factor. For instance, drinking at work or in public is generally more risky than drinking at home, where family members and familiar surroundings can keep a drinker out of trouble. Even drinking at home can be dangerous if combined with late-night smoking or hazardous household chores. It is especially dangerous to mix drinking and driving.

There are certain negative consequences of drinking that do depend almost exclusively on the amount of alcohol consumed. An example is the disabling and potentially fatal liver disease known as cirrhosis. In this disease the cells of the liver are poisoned by excessive exposure to alcohol. Increasing numbers of these cells become inflamed and die, leaving useless scar tissue.

Approximately 30,000 Americans die each year from advanced cirrhosis, and it is one of the leading causes of death among middle-aged men in much of the industrialized world. A large fraction of the victims of cirrhosis would not have contracted the disease if they did not drink. Among alcoholics who drink the equivalent of 10 drinks daily, 8 percent have cirrhosis and 25 percent have acutely inflamed livers, a precursor to cirrhosis. Furthermore, only half the people who die from cirrhosis would meet the main diagnostic criteria for alcoholism, although most of them are heavy drinkers. In actuarial terms, a person who has three to four drinks daily incurs some additional risk of liver injury. But generally a person has to drink very heavily for a number of years—probably 15 or more—before cirrhosis becomes not only a disability but a threat to life.

Another important type of alcohol-related death occurs in traffic accidents. Each year some 15 million people are involved in reported motor vehicle crashes in the United States, according to figures from the National Highway Traffic Safety Administration. In 1984 these crashes caused about 44,000 fatalities and over 3 million injuries. David Reed of Harvard University has calculated that approximately one quarter of these deaths and one tenth of these injuries are the direct result of intoxication, meaning that they would not have occurred if the drivers involved in the accidents had not been drinking (Chapter 3 discusses these findings in more detail). Perhaps another quarter of all traffic deaths involve alcohol in a more tangential way.

Traffic accidents receive the most attention, but as many people die each year from other kinds of accidents—especially falls, fires, and drownings—as on the nation's highways. People who die in these accidents do not routinely have their blood tested for the presence of alcohol, as is the case with traffic fatalities, so it is more difficult to accurately attribute a percentage of these accidents to drinking. But researchers have estimated that alcohol may be involved in as many as 40 percent of these accidents—the equivalent of over 20,000 deaths.

Alcohol-related overdoses are another major source of mortality. About 10,000 people die each year from this cause, half from alcohol alone, half from the combination of alcohol and other drugs. In the latter cases, death certificates list suicide as the cause of death about 40 percent of the time. Alcohol has an appallingly strong connection with suicide. One third of the nearly 30,000 suicides in the United States each year have alcohol in their blood at death. Among the 200,000 to 400,000 attempted suicides each year, alcohol problems are five times more common than in a comparable nonsuicidal group.

Homicides are another form of violent death that may be related to drunkenness. Each year about 10,000 murders occur in situations involving alcohol. However, as with suicides involving alcohol, it is impossible to unambiguously attribute these deaths to drinking, since so many other factors are invariably involved.

Fetal alcohol syndrome is a substantial medical problem caused by excessive maternal drinking during pregnancy. An estimated 500 to 1,000 of the infants born each year to alcoholic mothers are mentally handicapped due to fetal alcohol syndrome. Finally, there is a statistically uncertain contribution of alcohol abuse to deaths and disabilities due to head and neck cancers; cardiovascular diseases, especially stroke; diabetes; and

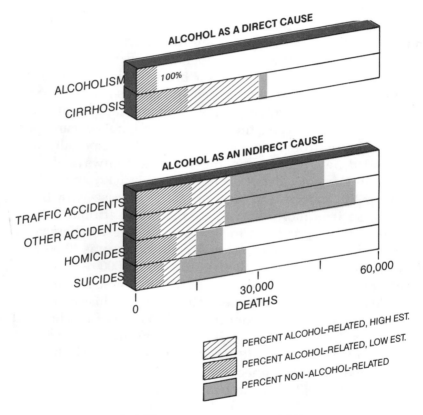

SELECTED CAUSES OF DEATH — U.S., 1975

FIGURE 1.3 The number of fatalities in the United States related to alcohol cannot be precisely determined, because of complicating factors and inadequate reporting networks. But various ranges for alcohol-related deaths can be estimated using data for a given year—in this case 1975. Sources: University of California, Social Research Group (Berkeley, California), National Center for Health Statistics.

organic brain syndromes. The presence of heavy smoking and other risk factors for these diseases among heavy drinkers complicates statistical analyses.

Adding up all of the fatalities related to excessive drinking, Dean Gerstein of the National Research Council concludes that alcohol may be involved in a maximum of 150,000 deaths per year (see Figure 1-3). Approximately 2 million people died in 1983 in the United States. Alcohol could therefore have been involved in about 1 out of every 13 deaths. This does not mean that 150,000 people would not die each year if they did not drink. But curtailing the abuse of alcohol would certainly prevent some of these deaths. "How much less is not certain," writes Gerstein, "but a figure in the area of 50,000 theoretically preventable deaths seems reasonable."

These are tragic statistics, and few people in the United States do not know someone who has been touched by them. But they are far from the whole picture. Fatalities are the most drastic consequences of alcohol abuse, but they also point to a much larger body of injuries, illnesses, psychological difficulties, and interpersonal problems related to alcohol.

Health care expenses are a partial indicator of these more widespread negative consequences of drinking. Estimates of problem drinkers in hospital populations run to 30 percent or more, and many diagnoses in hospitals could include secondary diagnoses of alcoholism or alcohol abuse. Medical expenditures required by alcohol abuse and alcoholism have been calculated at $10 to $20 billion per year, and estimates of lost productivity in the workplace tend to be much higher. These numbers are hard to pin down, since alcohol abuse is so often just one of several factors contributing to an illness. But there is widespread agreement that excessive drinking exacts a heavy toll on overall levels of health.

Another category of consequences known to be widespread but hard to quantify consists of the negative emotional effects of alcohol abuse. Many alcoholics report feeling depressed, anxious, powerless, or troubled. But all of these feelings also occur in people who don't drink. According to Gerstein, "Most of the behavioral and subjective states that we find easy to ascribe to drunkenness—sociability or sadness, daring or tranquillity, aggression or passivity—do not spring directly from the bottle but find expression due to the social circumstances and personalities in which drunkenness is brought into play."

The same complexities mark the link between alcohol and social relationships. Personal accounts make it clear that alcohol abuse can exacerbate family problems, mar work relationships, and limit or abort career opportunities. But social relationships are so complex that it is difficult to analyze the specific role of alcohol in shaping them. In many cases, drinking can act more as a justification or excuse for destructive behavior than as a root cause of that behavior.

The Positive Side of Drinking

No accounting of the consequences of alcohol consumption would be complete without mention of the positive aspects of drinking. As the National Research Council panel on alcohol abuse noted in its 1981 report, "That benefit results from drinking is usually conceded even by those who are most appalled by the damages. Over [$60 billion was spent in 1983] on alcohol by people who could have chosen to spend the money on better housing, new clothes, roast beef, or vacations." These expenditures on alcoholic beverages make a substantial contribution to the nation's economy.

The alcoholic beverage industry consists of three tiers: the distillers, vintners, and brewers; the distribution and importation companies; and the bars, taverns, liquor stores, groceries, restaurants, and other outlets that sell alcohol to the public. Many of these outlets depend on the sale of alcohol for their profit margins. Also, many spectator and participant sports have become closely linked with alcohol sales.

Another important consideration is the amount of drinking that does not lead to any serious trouble. Although some people regard any departure from sobriety as a deplorable social and moral problem, for most people short-lived periods of mild intoxication do not cause any substantial harm. Many people regard drinking and intoxication as relaxing and enjoyable, as a harmless indulgence, or as a way of turning an ordinary event into a festive occasion. Alcohol can also contribute to such positive family events as shared evening cocktails or celebratory toasts. "How do we quantify the effects of alcohol as parts of such occasions?" asks Gerstein. "On the basis of current data, we simply cannot do so. This does not make them any less real."

Moderate drinking may even have a positive effect on health in certain circumstances. A number of studies have suggested a statistical association between moderate consumption of alcohol and a reduced risk of ischemic heart disease[2], the leading cause of death in the United States. If the use of alcohol were responsible for even a 1 percent reduction in the net risk of coronary death, about 5,000 fewer people would die from this cause each year. However, these studies have only examined special groups of people and have disagreed on what level of consumption is protective. Efforts to find a biochemical mechanism responsible for this protection have so far been unsuccessful, and the possibility of significant unidentified variables exists. It may be that the benefits of moderate drinking are simply a reflection of the benefits of moderation as a personal style.

Relatively few researchers have concentrated on the beneficial effects of drinking, whether economic, social, or personal. They have been much more industrious in uncovering and quantifying its negative consequences. There can be no question that these consequences are severe. But as we begin in the next chapter to investigate policies that can reduce the number of problems associated with drinking, the positive consequences must be kept in mind. If the cost of curtailing alcohol problems is a marked reduction in the possible benefits of drinking, an initiative in that direction is unlikely to gain wide support.

---

[2]Ischemic heart disease refers to tissue damage caused by obstruction of the flow of arterial blood to the heart.

2

Why Prevention?

A N EXAMINATION OF CURRENT ATTITUDES and policies toward drinking reveals an intriguing gap in America's approach to alcohol-related problems. The past several decades have seen a great expansion of concern over the problem of alcoholism. As this concern has grown, many people have come to believe that most of the problems caused by alcohol occur within the relatively small group of people (1 to 4 percent of the adult population) who could be classified as alcoholics. It follows that the best way to deal with alcohol-related problems is to identify people who are or who are likely to become alcoholics and to treat them and those whom they put at greatest risk—namely their children and spouses—as effectively as possible. Volunteer organizations and medical programs have arisen to provide this treatment, and much of the public has come to understand and support such efforts.

This focus on alcoholism has undoubtedly improved the lives of some of America's most troubled drinkers and their families. It has directed attention toward a large part, perhaps the single largest part, of this country's alcohol problems, and it has dealt with those problems in interesting and productive ways. But alcoholics are not the only people who ever cause or get into trouble because of drinking. Certainly they are the drinkers most likely to experience physical or emotional distress because of alcohol. But the much greater number of more moderate drinkers can also suffer from the problems caused by drinking—the accidents, the illnesses, the marital discord. These are the people for whom certain kinds of prevention programs can be uniquely effective.

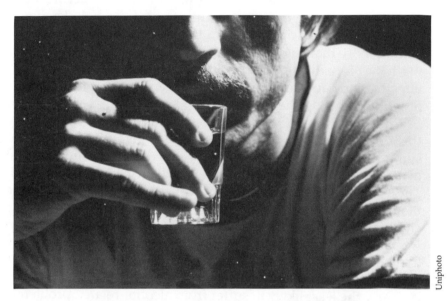

Heavy drinkers are not the only ones with problems. Anyone who drinks may at some time be prone to alcohol-related accidents, family conflict, and illnesses. Thus, treatment programs for people classified as alcoholics ameliorate only a portion of America's alcohol problems.

There are several ways to investigate the critical question of how alcohol-related problems are distributed across different kinds of drinkers. One is to examine how often people drink excessively. There are safer and less safe ways of drinking a given amount of alcohol. A person who drinks a little every night at home is less likely to get in a fight or an accident than a person who goes on binges in public twice a month. Both people may drink the same amount of alcohol overall, but the binge drinker is at greater risk during his or her infrequent nights on the town (although the stay-at-home drinker is of course not immune to alcohol problems).

A survey by Michael Polich and Bruce Orvis of personnel in the U.S. Air Force sheds some light on this important statistic.[1] The population they studied cannot be taken to represent the entire United States, but it is typical of the young, employed male population. Polich and Orvis divided the 3,078 people they surveyed into different categories of drinkers according to their overall average daily consumption of alcohol. They also noted how many times a year these different drinkers consumed more than eight drinks in a single day. Since little drinking took place during the day, these "intensive drinking days" effectively meant that the drinker was intoxicated for at least a few hours during the evening.

What Polich and Orvis found is revealing. The 4 percent of this population who were *very heavy* drinkers (those who consumed a daily average of 10 or more drinks) accounted for just over a quarter of the total number of drunk days experienced. The 23 percent who were *heavy* drinkers (each averaging more than two but fewer than ten drinks daily) generated about five eighths of the drunk days. The 57 percent of Air Force men who consumed an average of less than two drinks each day (the remaining 16 percent were abstainers) still generated one eighth of the drunk days. Individually, the last set of drinkers is clearly the least likely to suffer from alcohol-related problems, but there are so many of them that their potential contribution to the total problem adds up.

A more direct way to probe the distribution of alcohol-related problems is to ask survey respondents about past problems. In their survey, Polich and Orvis also gathered data about the number of serious incidents associated with alcohol for different kinds of drinkers. Again, they found that the very heavy drinkers accounted for only about one quarter of the total number of people with two or more serious incidents. A national household survey reported by Walter Clark and Lorraine Midanik confirmed these findings.[2] They found that the 11 percent of

[1] J. M. Polich and B. R. Orvis. *Alcohol Problems: Patterns and Prevalence in the U.S. Air Force.* Santa Monica, Calif.: Rand Corporation, 1979.

[2] W. B. Clark and L. Midanik. Results of the 1979 National Survey (mimeograph). Berkeley, Calif: Social Research Group, University of California, 1980.

all adults categorized as heavy drinkers (defined as people consuming an average of more than two drinks per day) suffered less than half of the total number of health and social problems associated with alcohol (see Figure 2-1).

These studies clearly indicate that alcohol-related problems occur *throughout* the drinking population. Even if America's 15 million heaviest drinkers were to stop drinking tomorrow, a substantial fraction of the country's alcohol problems would

ALCOHOL-RELATED PROBLEMS WITH

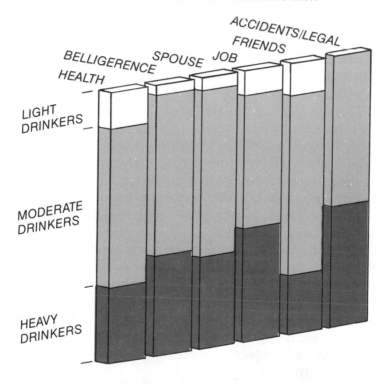

CONTRIBUTION OF DRINKERS TO REPORTED PROBLEMS

FIGURE 2.1 National surveys reveal that the majority of certain alcohol-related problems affect moderate drinkers—those having up to two drinks per day. Heavier drinkers are more likely to suffer some sort of alcohol problem than are moderate drinkers, but there are so many more moderate drinkers that their contribution to the total problem adds up. Source: University of California, Social Research Group (Berkeley, California).

remain. These problems are borne by relatively unexceptional drinkers. They are people who do not always drink excessively; they may just drink inappropriately, recklessly, or unluckily. As Mark Moore of Harvard University puts it, "The problem of ill-timed drunkenness, badly fit into the environment, generates a substantial portion of the medical problems, the violence and crime problems, the employment problems, and even the marital problems that involve alcohol. In other words, a large portion of the alcohol problem is created by people who would never think of themselves as problem drinkers." This situation has important implications for public policy.

The Elements of Prevention

If America is to reduce the number of alcohol-related problems that occur among people who are not alcoholics, it must consider diversifying its current approaches to drinking problems. Techniques drawn from the alcoholism perspective alone clearly cannot reach this widely distributed part of the problem. For one thing, it would be impossibly expensive to provide individually tailored treatment for the many millions of drinkers in America. It would also be inappropriate. Unlike the heaviest drinkers, more moderate drinkers are not individually at great risk of suffering from some sort of problem. They would resent being treated as if they were.

A better and more practical way to reach the entire population of drinkers is through policies that can be thought of as preventive. Prevention has a different starting point from that of treatment, though its ultimate goals are similar. In a treatment program, people who are alcoholics or who are closely related to alcoholics are identified and offered help. Their care involves personalized, face-to-face relationships with other individuals, often over a prolonged period.

The prevention measures discussed in this book generally operate in a different way. They are nonpersonalized approaches that act throughout the drinking population. They do not focus on specific people. Rather, they can come into play for anyone who drinks. They seek to change the incentives, opportunities, risks, and expectations that surround drinkers in society. Their objective is to alter drinking practices in the general population or to break the link between those practices and adverse consequences.

Because of the complexity of that link, prevention measures can be fashioned from a wide variety of materials. The most extreme measures are those that draw on the force of the law to discourage a particular kind of drinking behavior. Drunk driving, which is the subject of Chapter 3, is the foremost example of such a behavior. Minimum drinking ages, public drunkenness, and restrictions on sales to intoxicated customers are other areas in which the law plays a role. In all of these cases, however, legal action is only one of a broad range of preventive actions that can help reduce the problem. The combined influence of many preventive initiatives can have a much greater effect than can legal constraints alone.

The prevention initiatives considered in this book fall into three broad categories. The first category includes those actions that affect the price and availability of alcohol. Taxes on alcohol, minimum age requirements, restrictions on the numbers and hours of outlets, and the actions of servers all influence the ease of access to alcoholic beverages. By altering these conditions, it may be possible to affect not only how much people drink but also where, when, and how they drink, factors that can be just as important as overall consumption.

Chapters 4 and 5 consider this category of prevention. Chapter 4 examines the effect that the price of alcohol has on drinking and on drinking problems, especially among the heaviest drinkers. Chapter 5 discusses what commercial servers can do to see that the people they serve do not end up in trouble.

The second category of preventive measures includes actions that seek to alter drinking practices more directly through various forms of education and persuasion. These actions might take the form of radio, television, or newspaper messages that discuss unsafe or inappropriate drinking practices. They might also consist of formal educational programs in the schools. Legal sanctions fall into this category, since the law is a particularly strong form of persuasion. The government can also try to set an example of drinking practices through its own actions and statements.

Chapters 6 and 7 explore some of these possibilities. Chapter 6 considers the important issue of drinking by young people, asking how education and other influences can mold their experiences with alcohol. Chapter 7 examines the role of the mass media in shaping drinking practices, through educational campaigns, advertising, and commercial programming.

The third category includes those actions that make the world a safer place in which to drink. These actions can involve both the physical and the social world. Changes in the physical world might mean safer homes, workplaces, consumer products, machines, and highways. Changes in the social environment might entail offering to drive an intoxicated person home from a party or a bar. Such possibilities are the subject of Chapter 8.

Not all of these strategies are guaranteed to work. As observed in Chapter 4, higher prices for alcohol have been found to reduce overall levels of consumption, traffic fatalities, and cirrhosis of the liver. Teaching people to drink safely and making the environment safer for drinking have less empirical backing. Nevertheless, each of these measures holds enough promise to be carefully considered.

It would also be a mistake to view a single prevention initiative outside of the full context of prevention. Each initiative draws strength from the others. Of course, each will fail or succeed only as it is implemented properly and thoroughly. But broad, comprehensive programs incorporating many different approaches are more likely to be successful than actions taken in isolation.

This perspective on alcohol-related problems requires that people resist the temptation to think in terms of opposed pairs: prohibition versus unlimited access, treatment versus prevention, education versus law enforcement. Says Moore, "I have a general kind of view that all of these things turn out to be more complementary than we are inclined to think, that public and private work together, that punitive and treatment approaches work together, that taxation and education work together, that all of the things that we imagine as being starkly opposite, as representing alternative routes, gain power when we put them together."

Considerations in Designing Prevention Policies

In deciding whether and how to implement preventive measures, policymakers and other concerned individuals must move intelligently. To be effective, instruments of prevention should reach a broad segment of the population. But any particular approach, if stretched too far, can become ineffective or even destructive. When prevention begins to infringe excessively on innocuous or beneficial aspects of drinking, it has the potential to do more harm than good.

Some people object to prevention on broader grounds, seeing any governmental attempt to influence drinking as an unwarranted restriction on personal freedom. In this view, governments should constrain a person's actions only when those actions could harm someone who is unable to protect himself. Risks that people take of their own accord, such as excessive drinking, should not be the concern of government.

Safeguarding individual freedoms, however, is not the only charge of government. Governments have also been seen as forces to enhance the general welfare, promote the spread of knowledge, and encourage civil behavior. The view that the government should promote good health has been gaining strength, as demonstrated by the antismoking and physical fitness campaigns. Of course, it is a moralistic position for the government to contend that people should act in such a way as to stay healthy. But it is a stance that the government has been encouraged to take.

Preventive measures may also augment personal freedoms by avoiding some of the moralistic judgments involved in other approaches to alcohol problems. Specifically, by acting broadly throughout the population, they avoid labeling people as alcoholics. They do not have to answer what Moore calls "a central, bedeviling issue": Who is a problem drinker and who is not? "We are used to thinking that anyone who drinks and is having associated problems such as unemployment or social or medical problems is an alcoholic, a 'protoalcoholic,' or a 'near-alcoholic,' " says Moore. "Partly for that reason, anyone in the general population who gets drunk and is arrested or falls down stairs feels nervous about defining himself or herself as a 'problem drinker,' because that means he or she is an alcoholic or is destined to become one, with all the associated special misery and special treatment."

Another possible objection to prevention is that it will compete with other approaches to alcohol-related problems. For instance, people may feel that prevention will take money away from treatment programs that have taken years to establish, or that it will implicitly condone certain drinking practices. However, there are good reasons to believe that treatment and prevention would be complementary rather than competitive. Prevention programs do not cost a great deal of money. They involve taxation, regulation, and messages that can be used over and over. Even a major mass media campaign can reach large numbers of people at low per capita costs.

Prevention programs may also reduce the number of people in need of treatment. According to several major studies, efforts that succeed in influencing general drinking practices also influence the number of very heavy drinkers. If this is the case, altering drinking habits among the general population could reduce the number of people who drink excessively. In addition, prevention programs can shield these drinkers from the adverse consequences of drinking in ways that treatment programs cannot, and they can reach the majority of problem drinkers who never do seek treatment.

Barriers to Prevention

Besides the general objections to prevention mentioned above, there are certain more pragmatic problems that often arise when considering prevention policies. As Margaret Hastings of the Illinois Commission on Mental Health and Developmental Disabilities says, "Prevention is a public health ideal that everyone favors—in the abstract. But when it comes to voting on real programs and real dollars, prevention policy has certain politically difficult characteristics."

For one thing, prevention is oriented toward the future. Its success is measured not in terms of immediate accomplishments but long-term goals. "It requires a commitment to future outcomes, not short-term results," says Hastings. "This is antithetical to an American political need attached to short electoral cycles: the need to show immediate gains. Elected officials have a hard time voting for prevention programs unless there is a well-educated constituency willing to keep those programs alive by reelecting leaders who support future-oriented policies."

Prevention can suffer from the lack of a well-defined constituency. Other health care lobbies concerned with such conditions as blindness, heart disease, and cancer have specific constituencies that foster state and national legislation. But "prevention cuts across categories," says Hastings. "It is a comprehensive concept, not a casualty area. This absence of a specific casualty constituency can act as an obstacle politically. Although prevention efforts may be seen as humane and cost-effective, they have trouble moving to the forefront of national, state, and local health and human services policy."

Finally, prevention policies almost invariably involve a conflict of values. People's attitudes toward alcohol are an obvious example. Many people see drinking as fundamentally immoral or, at least, morally weak. Others view drinking as a sign of liberal values or as a traditional means of sociability. The clash between these two outlooks can stymie political decision making, leaving prevention initiatives paralyzed. "In my seven years of experience in developing state policy," says Hastings, "the potential collision of values has been the major hurdle, and it grows more complicated as our belief systems become more pluralistic. Enormous pressures on legislators from individual industries, religions, and special interest groups make consensus difficult. These pressure groups often have far more influence on policy than their actual numbers of supporters would suggest."

Despite these practical obstacles to prevention, preventive measures have made considerable political headway in recent years, in large part because of the tremendous outpouring of support and action now focused on them. As William Mayer, former head of the Alcohol, Drug Abuse, and Mental Health Administration, says, "The extent and quality of attention now being directed toward alcohol-related problems is without precedent in our lifetimes. States, local areas, and the private sector at all levels are giving attention in new ways to alcohol-related problems that have had such debilitating effects on our society, effects that have for so long been denied. Alcohol abuse and alcoholism are now being recognized here and throughout the world as major public health problems, and prevention has a high priority. . . . Examples include the Presidential Commission on Drunk Driving, the Department of Health and Human Services' Secretarial Initiative on teenage alcohol abuse, and the enormous relative increases in the 1983 and 1984 federal research budget for alcohol abuse and alcoholism, which far outstripped increases for research in other health areas."

At the same time, many nongovernmental grass roots organizations have sprung up to combat the problem of drunk driving, including Mothers Against Drunk Driving (MADD), Remove Intoxicated Drivers (RID), and Students Against Drunk Driving (SADD). These groups have supported such preventive actions as increasing the drinking age, changing criminal penalties, and installing new classroom curricula.

Many other organizations in the United States also have the potential to make a significant contribution to the overall goal of reducing the number of alcohol problems. Just as prevention has diverse targets, so it can originate from diverse sources. Elected officials, treatment providers, business leaders, bureaucrats, volunteer groups, educators, churches, and many other individuals can act to implement the general idea of prevention, just as they have acted in the past to deal with alcoholism. Moreover, widespread public sentiment in the United States in favor of moderate drinking ensures a supportive climate for such efforts.

To give one example of unused potential, many government agencies not explicitly concerned with alcohol policy could play an important role in prevention. According to James Mosher and Joseph Mottl of the University of California at Berkeley, "Significant portions of federal authority to regulate the availability of alcohol and to respond to alcohol-related problems rest with federal agencies not usually associated with alcohol policy [such as the National Park Service, the Department of Defense, and the Internal Revenue Service]. This has resulted in little or no coordination in the development of the federal response to alcohol, particularly in the area of prevention. In some cases, contradictory policies are being made and enforced; in others, promising new prevention strategies (and potential new allies) are not being pursued."

The Need for Cooperation

For prevention to continue to make progress, the diverse range of groups and individuals with a stake in prevention need to cooperate and coordinate their efforts. Because prevention is a comprehensive concept, many different initiatives will be going on simultaneously. Information about the effectiveness of these initiatives, and about the practical difficulties of implementing them, must be shared if the initiatives are to survive and prosper. "This requires an unusual willingness to set priorities, share responsibilities, and believe in causes beyond a single individual, agency, or organizational turf," says Hastings.

Organizations and individuals may even cooperate to the extent of forming coalitions that can back prevention initiatives in local, state, and federal governments. Michael Fox of the Ohio General Assembly, who has had extensive experience building such coalitions, believes that they are a uniquely effective way to foster prevention policies:

Policy objectives and public polls have to be translated into coalitions, which can be built on diverse bases. Revenue is one common concern. Another is the rising cost of health care. A third is criminal legislation; chiefs of police, local sheriffs, fraternal orders of police, judges, and so forth are very interested in penal legislation. There is tremendous coalition-building potential over the concern about young people's involvement with alcohol. The opportunity to greatly expand government partnerships with the private sector, with respect to alcohol and substance abuse, has never been better. The visibility given this issue by groups like MADD and by campaigns to make the public aware of the social costs and consequences of the abuse of this product has created an opportunity to move and move quickly.

If you can design a coordinated strategy to incorporate all these factors, you will have built the base, the numbers, the power to confront opposing forces in the legislature. Now is the time to gather banners that have not traditionally been used together as effectively as they could be. I do not know how long the opportunity for building coalitions will last, but I suggest that this opening be used to the fullest extent to create prevention-oriented public policy.

3

Preventing Drunk Driving

D RUNK DRIVING IS AN EXCELLENT EXAMPLE of both the need and the opportunity for prevention to be comprehensive. Clearly, laws against drunk driving, enforced by the police and adjudicated by the courts, must play a leading role in the effort to keep people from driving while drunk. But legal action alone cannot solve the problem. Many other strategies also have the potential to significantly reduce drunk driving. Together with the law, these strategies can have a major effect.

There can be no question that alcohol is a major contributor to the problem of traffic safety in the United States. In about half of the 44,000 fatalities caused by traffic accidents in 1984, the drivers or other people killed in the accident had alcohol in their blood (see Figure 3-1). But this statistic can be misleading. It does not mean that if no one ever drove after drinking, highway fatalities would be cut in half. As David Reed of Harvard University points out, "Drinking-driving countermeasures can be legitimate and useful government actions, but . . . even if such countermeasures were perfectly successful, the savings in lives, injuries, and property loss would be less than widely quoted figures would lead one to believe."

The reason, explains Reed, is that the presence of alcohol in an accident does not always mean that alcohol caused the ac-

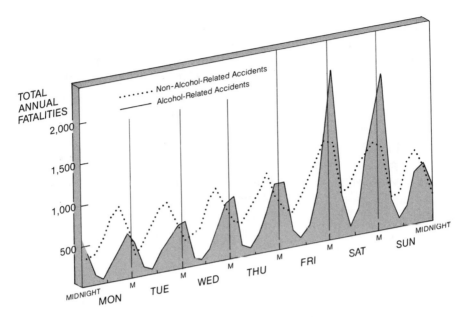

FIGURE 3.1   Traffic deaths occur more often in the evening and nighttime hours, when visibility is poor and drivers tend to be tired. Alcohol-related traffic fatalities are nearly twice as numerous on Friday and Saturday nights as on other nights, and they tend to peak a few hours later than fatalities that do not involve alcohol. Source: National Highway Traffic Safety Administration.

cident. In many accidents that kill people who have been drinking, the alcohol plays a minor or insignificant role. Roadside testing by researchers has shown that an average of 10 to 20 percent of all drivers on the road have measurable levels of alcohol in their blood. It is inevitable that some of these people will be involved in fatal accidents, even if their drinking is not to blame.

Using several epidemiological studies of drunk driving, Reed has calculated a more accurate estimate of the number of deaths that could be prevented if no one ever drove after drinking. These studies compared the blood alcohol levels of drivers involved in accidents with the blood alcohol levels of drivers not involved in accidents (this latter control group was randomly selected at times and places similar to those at which the accidents occurred). The data show that 24 percent of the fatalities would not have occurred if the drivers had not been drinking. Similar calculations give average estimates of 12 percent for the number of disabling injuries that would be prevented and 6 percent for the amount of preventable property damage. Of course, these figures are only estimates. Several factors that could not be included in the calculations could force these percentages higher or lower, and the data are far from perfect.

Nevertheless, these findings suggest that the number of theoretically preventable deaths, while not the 50 percent often cited, is still high. Nationwide, a 24 percent decrease in fatalities would mean that over 10,000 of the nearly 45,000 people killed annually in traffic accidents in recent years would not have died. Similarly, the number of theoretically preventable disabling injuries (the most ambiguous category) is between 150,000 and 300,000 per year, Reed estimates, and the property damage that could be prevented is over $1 billion. These figures indicate what might be possible. The question then becomes, how can the United States move toward these goals?

Do More Arrests Have an Effect?

The law in the United States (and throughout the world) clearly declares that people should not drive while drunk. Generally, legal codes specify a blood alcohol content (BAC) of between 0.08 and 0.10 percent, past which a person is legally intoxicated. Almost everyone agrees that drunk driving is reckless, therefore dangerous, and therefore wrong. Here, then, is a case where the law reinforces widely held public opinions.

The effectiveness of these laws, however, must be open to question. For every arrest made for driving while intoxicated (DWI), an estimated 500 to 2,000 drunk driving incidents go unpenalized, although more arrests are made for drunk driving in America than for any other offense and significant sums are spent on enforcement. Even doubling or quadrupling the number of arrests would leave the chance of arrest extremely small. With the possibility of getting caught so slim, it may seem that people would shrug off an effort by police to make more arrests.

Surprisingly, several studies show that this is not the case. An increased risk of arrest can significantly reduce drunk driving. The classic example is the British Road Safety Act of 1967. This act defined driving with a blood alcohol content of 0.08 to be an offense. The BAC was to be determined by an "Alcotest" breathalyzer device, one million of which were purchased by the British government. Police asked drivers to submit to the test given a reasonable cause, such as a road accident, a moving violation, or erratic driving. If the driver refused, illegal intoxication was assumed. Judges had no discretion in sentencing. The first offense resulted in a mandatory one-year suspension of a driver's license.

The Road Safety Act had a dramatic impact on Britain's drivers. In the three months after it took effect, traffic fatalities dropped 23 percent in Britain. In the first year of the act, the percentage of drivers killed who were legally drunk dropped from 27 percent to 17 percent.

These general trends mask several specific changes in British drinking practices. Research showed that the act did not significantly change the amount people in Britain drank. Rather, the act seems to have affected a very narrow slice of behavior— the custom of driving to and from pubs, especially on weekend nights. After the act took effect, many regular customers took to walking to pubs. Pub owners raised a considerable outcry, and a number of less conveniently located pubs closed.

Unfortunately, the successes of the act were relatively short-lived. Within a few years, traffic fatalities again began to climb. By 1973 the percentage of drivers killed who were drunk was back to its pre-1967 level. By 1975, for reasons still unknown, this percentage had risen to 36 percent, considerably above what it was before the act.

This evaporation of progress is a common feature of efforts to increase the risk of arrest. The usual explanation for it is that drivers eventually realize that the chances of arrest and punishment are not all that high. "People lose interest," says Charles Crawford, vice-president of the Ernest and Julio Gallo Winery. "The police lose interest, the judges have no more room to throw people in jail, and they start to forget about it." In the case of the British Road Safety Act, much of its initial effectiveness seems to have come from the breathalyzer, which had never been used in Britain before. The British expected the Alcotest to revolutionize the workings of the court on drunk driving cases. A scientific mechanism would replace the old system of patrols and trials. In fact, the breathalyzer had no such effect. Well-publicized cases soon established narrow limits to its authority. Standards for its use took several years to develop, and British police used it less frequently than did police in other countries. As the respect for and fear of the Alcotest declined, so did the effectiveness of the act.

Several drunk driving programs in the United States have produced results similar to those of the British Road Safety Act. In the 1970s the Department of Transportation funded 35 locally organized and managed Alcohol Safety Action Projects in various parts of the country. Each project sought in its own way to combine an increased risk of arrest, more effective trial and rehabilitation procedures, and public education to reduce the number of accidents caused by drunk driving. By increasing surveillance, targeting patrols for specific times and places, and motivating police to make arrests, many of the jurisdictions involved were able to double and triple the number of DWI arrests.

The studies that attempted to evaluate these local projects suffered from serious methodological flaws, including noncomparable sites, inadequate controls, and a premature expansion of the program. But in their final report, the projects' national evaluators found that 12 of the 35 had produced a discernible effect on nighttime auto fatalities—a good indicator of drunk driving. These 12 projects reduced fatalities an average of 30 percent over three years, which is broadly comparable to the 23 percent reduction in fatalities noted in the British program. Independent researchers, however, have concluded that the positive effects were much smaller.

The overall conclusion that can be drawn from the various drunk driving studies is that an increased risk of arrest does deter drunk driving. The National Research Council panel on alcohol abuse concludes that "some moderately persuasive evidence exists suggesting that effectively enforced drunken driving laws will deter drunken driving and reduce accidents and

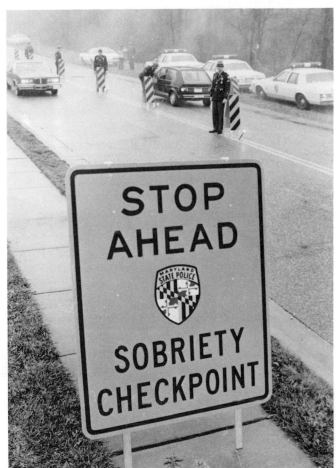

Roadblocks are a particularly controversial method used by police forces to increase their surveillance of drivers and to deter drunk driving.

fatalities associated with it." Increased police surveillance is especially important at night, when most alcohol-induced traffic fatalities occur. Moreover, recent studies have shown that the speed with which drunk driving cases are decided in court can substantially influence the effectiveness of new drunk driving laws. However, other research questions remain to be answered to determine how best to reinforce the ongoing shift of attitudes toward drunk driving.

Finally, increasing the risk of arrest is apt to be costly. For example, the Alcohol Safety Action Projects cost $88 million, not counting the costs of state and local enforcement, the expense of treatment programs borne by those arrested, and the social costs of increased police surveillance. At the most these projects saved 563 lives, for an average minimum cost of $156,000 per life saved. Many other traffic safety improvements have the potential to save lives more cost-effectively, according to the Department of Transportation, though they may not be able to save as many lives as increased enforcement of drunk driving laws.

Do Tougher Penalties Have an Effect?

There may be another way besides increased enforcement to keep people from driving while drunk. If the penalties imposed by courts and juries for drunk driving are severe, people may think twice about taking to the road when intoxicated. This alternative has the potential to be less costly than increased police surveillance, except for the drunk drivers caught, and would also concentrate the burden of stricter laws on drunk drivers rather than on all drivers.

The prime example of harsh penalties for drunk driving is found in the Scandinavian countries. There a first DWI offense commonly results in imprisonment, fines of up to 10 percent of a person's after-tax income, or license suspensions exceeding one year. Anecdotal evidence indicates that these tough penalties are effective deterrents, but social science research has been unable to uncover any hard proof.

Research has also shown that efforts to impose tougher penalties in America have not had much effect. In part, this seems to be caused by people's belief that "it can't happen to me." "After all," Reed observes, "those who currently drive drunk are not deterred by the small risk of a very severe penalty— accidental death."

Even when a drunk driver is brought to trial, judges, juries, and even police and prosecutors are often reluctant to impose tough penalties on DWI offenders. "Many people in our society do not view driving after drinking as deviant behavior," observes Reed. "If the general feeling of the public is, 'There but for the grace of God go I,' it is doubtful that severe penalties will be applied often even if they are authorized by law." However, the recent tendency of state legislatures to toughen drunk driving laws may indicate that these attitudes are changing.

The reluctance to impose harsh penalties may also stem from confusion over the nature of the offense. Mass media ads may have caused part of the problem. Some ads have suggested that any level of drinking is dangerous when combined with driving. If this were true, 75 percent of the population would have broken the law, since this is the proportion of people who in one national survey admit to having driven after drinking. If people feel they have broken the law themselves, they are inclined to judge others leniently.

In fact, the offense is *drunken* driving. Many people who drink and drive are not legally intoxicated, though their driving may be impaired. If these people knew how much a person had to drink to be convicted, they might be more willing to convict others of the crime. To be considered intoxicated in most states, a person who has not recently eaten typically has to have four to five drinks within an hour (although this amount varies greatly for different people). A typical BAC for a DWI offender who is brought to trial is 0.15 percent, which would require a small person to consume six to seven drinks in an hour on an empty stomach. Most Americans have probably never driven with this much alcohol in their blood.

Finally, tougher penalties for drunk driving bring their own costs, in addition to the costs imposed on the people who are caught. The length of trials and number of appeals are both likely to rise, further burdening an overtaxed court system. If drunk drivers are to be given jail terms, the expense of their imprisonment also has to be taken into account.

Despite such drawbacks, it is clear that police surveillance and appropriate penalties must be a component of society's effort to deal with drunk driving, and the use of these legal sanctions has been increasing in recent years. As the panel concludes, "At a minimum, [drunk driving laws] help sustain a widely shared disapprobation of drunken driving. They also provide an opportunity to attack a given drinking practice more aggressively if the society is willing to commit the resources, publicity, and attention necessary to make deterrence a social phenomenon rather than an abstract concept."

As noted at the beginning of this chapter, however, legal sanctions are not the sole answer to the problem of drunk driving. Many other preventive measures can also keep people from driving when drunk. The remaining chapters in this book describe these measures in detail and present the evidence for their effectiveness. The rest of this chapter outlines the main features of these measures, noting in particular their relevance to drunk driving.

Price and Availability of Alcohol

As described in Chapter 4, research has shown that higher prices for alcohol can significantly reduce the amount that people drink. Price-induced decreases in consumption have in turn been linked to declines in the incidence of drunk driving and cirrhosis of the liver. For the past three decades, the price of alcohol has been falling with respect to the price of other goods. A substantial part of this decline is due to federal and state taxes on alcohol not having kept up with inflation. Thus, the government may be able to reduce drunk driving by raising its taxes on alcohol.

It is difficult to quantify exactly how much less drunk driving would occur if taxes on alcohol were to rise. There are also economic and social costs associated with raising alcohol taxes. Nevertheless, this is a good example of how changes in general drinking practices can influence drunk driving.

It may also be possible to reduce drunk driving through specific steps affecting the availability of alcohol. Since World War II, restrictions on alcohol sales have gradually been weakening. Alcoholic beverages have been sold in more and more places, those places have been open longer hours, and minimum drinking ages in many states have gone down (although recently they have begun to go back up). Evidence from the United States that a greater number of outlets selling alcohol causes more drinking is still inconclusive. But several studies have indicated that a lower minimum drinking age does lead to greater accident and fatality rates among young people who have been drinking (Chapter 6). As the panel writes, "There is reasonable evidence that prohibition for youths does have some effect on their drinking and in particular that the choice of a minimum drinking age has a small but consistently exacerbating effect on the auto accident and fatality rates."

Another way to change the availability of alcohol is to have the people who serve alcohol, whether bartenders or private hosts, see to it that their customers or guests do not have too much to drink and then try to drive home (Chapter 5). In over half the states in the nation, "dramshop" laws impose this responsibility on commercial servers by making them liable for the damage done by underage or "obviously intoxicated" patrons to whom they serve alcoholic beverages. These laws are not as effective as they might be, however, because of the vagueness of the term "obviously intoxicated" and because they offer little guidance to servers on how to avoid liability.

In recent years, interest has been building in ways to make these laws more effective. One suggestion has been to broaden these laws to recognize a server's overall level of responsibility. If servers had standards of practice to follow in their business, courts or legislators could absolve servers who followed those standards from the liability for damage caused by patrons who drive drunk despite the server's efforts.

Educational Campaigns

Another approach to preventing drunk driving is through educational campaigns employing the mass media or local organizations such as hospitals, churches, and schools. These campaigns enjoy considerable prestige in the United States and have the potential to reach millions of people. As discussed in Chapter 7, however, evidence for their effectiveness remains scanty. People already know that drunk driving is dangerous and agree that the police and courts should move effectively to deal with it. Moreover, it is unlikely that educational campaigns will be powerful enough to fundamentally alter a person's beliefs about drinking, which are set by the entire social environment, including peer groups and family.

But there is one kind of educational campaign that holds more promise. This approach, which has been tried less often, is to teach people ways to avoid driving when dangerously or illegally drunk. It might include personal rules of thumb for knowing how much alcohol one can drink before reaching a certain BAC level, self-administered sobriety tests, or alternatives to driving when one has had too much to drink.

Of course, such information would have to exist for it to be disseminated, and increased research is needed on such matters. But even where usable findings are available, a serious problem remains. Mass media campaigns invariably shy away from any suggestion that people might drive after drinking, whether that drinking results in drunkenness or not. To hint that people might drive after drinking even though they are not legally drunk might be seen as encouraging this behavior. For example, writes Reed, "It is known that drowsiness, one of the obvious effects of drinking, impairs driving ability, yet public information and education campaigns from government and private sources consistently omit such suggestions as taking caffeine, driving with the windows open, or playing the radio when driving after drinking (although it is frequently and accurately pointed out that coffee does not reverse the intoxicating effects of alcohol). Presumably, such suggestions are omitted because they could be perceived as encouraging drunk driving by lowering its expected costs." This problem of possibly encouraging driving after drinking will surface again in the section below on reducing environmental risk.

If an educational campaign about drunk driving were instituted, certain kinds of media could be especially effective. Charles Crawford suggests putting several pages on the effects of alcohol in driver's license handbooks, which are among the most widely read booklets in America. "If every driver's handbook had a few pages, not on punitive laws but on what causes drunk driving and what constitutes social responsibility, I think it would mean a lot," he says.

Changing the Environment

Laws, server intervention, and mass media campaigns are designed to reduce the amount of drunk driving and hence the number of accidents caused by it. But it may also be possible to reduce the risk associated with drunk driving, regardless of how often people do it.

As discussed in Chapter 8, the most efficient physical devices now available to make driving safer are passive restraints, including automatic seat belts and air bags. These devices would be more effective for drunk drivers than for sober drivers, because studies show that drunk drivers involved in accidents are less likely to use conventional seat belts than are all drivers involved in accidents. Similarly, changes in road designs to make roads less confusing or distracting would help drunk drivers even more than sober drivers, since the ability to divide attention among tasks is one of the first capacities to diminish when people drink.

Another possibility is to equip cars with devices that detect an intoxicated driver and keep the car from starting or make it very conspicuous, say, by flashing its lights or honking the horn. Several such devices have been suggested. One is an analyzer that would sniff the air around a driver's head for any trace of alcohol. Another would detect errors characteristic of drinking, such as oversteering. There are also various kinds of skills testers, such as one that requires drivers to punch random numbers into a keyboard.

Of course, drivers could disconnect any such device or have someone else take the test for them. Even so, these devices could have the important effect. They could remind a driver and anyone else whose aid was enlisted that he or she was about to do a dangerous thing. The general public would probably object to the inconvenience, annoyance, and cost of having such devices in all cars. But they could be installed in the cars of select groups, such as people who have been arrested for drunk driving before.

Conclusions

To deal effectively with drunk driving, society must approach the problem from many different directions simultaneously. Beefed-up surveillance and tougher penalties for drunk drivers are two approaches that must be part of the solution. Drunk drivers kill and injure enough innocent third parties to warrant legal intervention, and Americans generally agree that drunk drivers should be arrested and punished.

At the same time, there are many other preventive options that should not be overlooked in an effort to get tough with drunk drivers. Higher taxes on alcohol, changes in the drinking age, responsible oversight by servers, educational campaigns, safer cars and highways, and steps to deal with repeat offenders all have at least a theoretical capability to reduce drunk driving. As we will see in the remaining chapters of this book, there are advantages and disadvantages to each of these steps, and the evidence for their effectiveness is not always conclusive. But as part of a broad, comprehensive program of prevention, they have the potential to make a significant and lasting difference.

4

The Price and Availability of Alcohol

FOR OVER THREE DECADES the average price of alcoholic beverages in relation to that of other commodities has been going down. One of the main reasons for this decline is that federal and state taxes on alcohol have not kept up with inflation. Federal taxes on beer and wine have not changed since 1951, when they were set at 16 cents on a six-pack of beer and from 3 to 67 cents on a 750-milliliter bottle of wine. Federal taxes on distilled liquors did not change from 1951 until 1984, when they rose from $1.68 on a fifth of 80 proof liquor to $1.92. State taxes on alcoholic beverages have risen gradually during this period, but not at anywhere near the rate of inflation.

Thus, the "real" price of alcohol—its price relative to that of other goods and services — has dropped steadily (see Figure 4.1). Since 1967, inflation has cut the real price of distilled liquors nearly in half. The real prices of beer and wine have dropped by about a quarter and a fifth, respectively. Alcoholic beverages are now so inexpensive that their prices are within range of many nonalcoholic drinks. "Soft drinks and beer now sell at roughly the same price," says Dan Beauchamp of the University of North Carolina. "This was not true 15 years ago. The cost of nonalcoholic beverages has more than tripled in the same

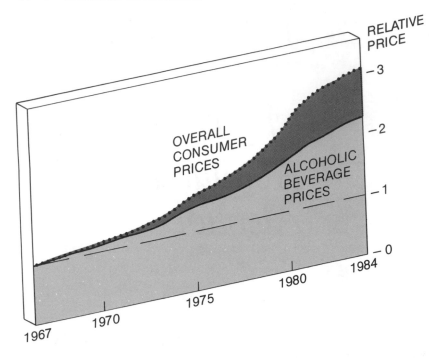

FIGURE 4.1 The average price of alcoholic beverages has not been going up as fast as the average price of all goods and services. As a result, alcoholic beverages have become relatively cheaper, which accounts for part of the rise in consumption over the past several decades. Source: Bureau of Labor Statistics, U.S. Department of Labor.

period that the cost of alcoholic beverages has less than doubled, and we now see price convergence of the two."

During the last three and a half decades, the per capita consumption of alcohol has been on the rise. It stayed roughly the same in the 1950s, spurted up in the 1960s, and rose slowly in the 1970s and 1980s. Since 1950, the per capita consumption of alcohol has risen over 30 percent.

One cannot assume that all of this increased consumption came about because alcoholic beverages were getting cheaper. Other factors, such as higher incomes, changing health habits, more tolerant attitudes toward drinking, and expanded marketing efforts may also have come into play. However, research to determine the weight of these competing factors relative to price changes was not widely conducted in this period.

Still, several lines of experimental and econometric evidence indicate that the price of alcohol has a substantial effect on how much people drink, which means that federal and state governments, by not keeping taxes up with inflation, have contributed to the increase in drinking in America since the 1950s. Similarly, it means that federal and state governments, by increasing their taxes on alcohol, have the capability to reduce the consumption of alcohol in this country. To decide whether they should do so requires a careful balancing of the costs of raising taxes against the costs of the alcohol-related problems that could be eliminated by reducing drinking.

Price is not the only attribute of alcohol sales that governments can control. There are a host of ways in which alcohol can become more or less available: New outlets or new kinds of outlets can open in neighborhoods or shopping centers; bars or liquor stores can keep longer hours; the minimum drinking age can go down or up. All of these changes can influence how easy it is to get alcohol and how much or where people drink. They are all potential instruments of public policies aimed at preventing alcohol problems.

Recent decades have seen a general relaxation of restrictions on the availability of alcohol. More outlets have opened, and they have been open more hours of the day. Drinking ages have gone down (although in some states they have more recently increased). The real price of alcohol has fallen. Given the toll that drinking exacts on society, many people have begun to ask whether it is possible to reenergize this gradually weakening regulatory apparatus to reduce the number of alcohol-related problems in America.

Government Regulation of Alcohol Sales

Throughout American history commerce in alcoholic beverages has been closely regulated and heavily taxed by federal and state governments. The first internal revenue law enacted by Congress under the Constitution was a liquor excise tax. Until Prohibition, taxes on alcohol were a major source of income for the federal government. In 1907 they constituted 80 percent of all federal internal tax revenues. Even at the beginning of World War II they accounted for 10 percent of these revenues. Today they figure very lightly in governmental budgets, averaging only about 1 percent of revenues at the federal, state, and local levels.

The repeal of Prohibition did not signal the end of governmental attempts to control alcohol. On the contrary, a host of federal, state, and local agencies oversee the commerce of alcohol from manufacture through final sale. At the federal level, the Bureau of Alcohol, Tobacco, and Firearms licenses manufacturers, wholesalers, and importers and regulates the advertising, size of containers, potency, and labeling of alcoholic beverages. It also collects around $5.5 billion each year from taxes on alcohol, with state and local governments taking another $6 billion (on total retail sales of over $60 billion).

Other federal agencies also have an influence on the price and availability of alcohol. The Department of Defense controls alcohol sales in clubs and post exchanges throughout the military. Eight million people are eligible to buy alcohol at these outlets, making this jurisdiction larger than that of many states. The Small Business Administration, since changing its rules in the late 1960s, has been lending money to the owners of taverns and liquor stores. And, as of this writing, the Internal Revenue Service's rulings on deductions for business-related meals and drinks countenance the three-martini lunch.

State and local governments have an even more prominent role in regulating the alcoholic beverage industry. They control almost every aspect of retail sale. All states set a minimum age for legal purchase, ranging from 18 to 21 years, and prescribe penalties for retailers who knowingly sell to underage customers. Most states restrict advertising, hours of sale, selling on credit, and so forth. The 21st Amendment left it to the states to decide if they wanted to remain dry. Many states have passed this option to local jurisdictions. In 1983 about 8 million of the United States' 226 million people lived in dry jurisdictions.

After Prohibition, 18 states created state or county liquor monopolies, to separate private profit from at least parts of the industry. The other states and the District of Columbia created licensing systems in which a regulatory agency oversees the distribution and sale of alcoholic beverages. Known as Alcoholic Beverage Control (ABC) boards in most states, these agencies decide which wholesalers and retailers will be permitted to operate in the state. They can also influence the density, location, and kind of retail outlets through their licensing activities. Finally, these boards license outlets such as restaurants that sell alcohol for on-site consumption.

The ABC boards were originally established to prevent the abuses of the pre-Prohibition era. They were intended to curb vicious or excessive drinking. But this purpose has gradually faded. A survey conducted in the mid-1970s by Medicine in the Public Interest found that the overwhelming majority of ABC administrators felt their responsibilities were not in any way related to public health.[1] They instead stressed the importance of collecting tax revenues, maintaining orderly markets, and excluding crime from the business.

Yet it is clear that ABC laws also promote temperance and discourage inappropriate drinking, albeit less visibly. Minimum age laws, limits on the number and nature of outlets, and to some extent high taxes are all intended to limit the availability of alcohol and reduce the harm of inappropriate drinking. Recently, interest has been growing in again strengthening these mechanisms to lessen drinking problems. But the ghost of Prohibition continues to restrain such preventive efforts. It would be an important step forward to dissociate these efforts from the distorted image of Prohibition that now prevails.

*Alcohol Prices, Highway Fatalities, and
Cirrhosis Death Rates*

A fundamental law of economics holds that as the price of something goes up, people will generally buy less of it. This undoubtedly explains part of the decline in drinking during Prohibition. The price of alcohol roughly tripled or quadrupled after the 18th Amendment took effect. Many people, especially

---

[1]Medicine in the Public Interest. *The Effects of Alcoholic-Beverage-Control Laws.* Washington, D.C.: Medicine in the Public Interest, Inc., 1979.

those with lower incomes, could not afford to drink as much as they had before, even if they had access to alcohol.

The same effect, in reverse, may also account for part of the increase in per capita consumption that has occurred since the 1950s (see Figure 4-2). Over that period the real price of alcohol has dropped, largely because federal and state taxes have not kept up with inflation. At the same time, per capita consumption has gone up over 30 percent.

Of course, different people respond to changes in the price of alcohol in different ways. If a tax increase were to up the price of alcohol, one person might buy less, another might

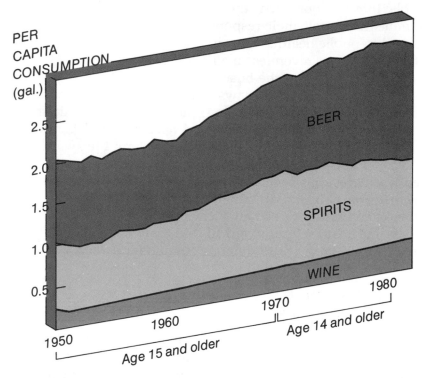

FIGURE 4.2 The per capita consumption of alcohol by adults in the United States has risen over 30 percent since 1950, with the greatest increase occurring during the 1960s. A number of factors have contributed to this increased consumption, including lower relative prices, more liberal attitudes toward drinking, and higher personal incomes. Source: National Institute on Alcohol Abuse and Alcoholism.

switch to a cheaper brand, another might drink just as much as before and pay the extra cost. This uncertain behavior is especially critical in the case of heavy drinkers, who account for a substantial portion of all alcohol consumed.

But even though it is difficult to predict how a particular person will behave, it is possible to draw conclusions about large groups of people. For instance, a tenfold increase during World War I in the price of aquavit in Denmark (the national beverage at that time) greatly reduced per capita consumption and the prevalence of heavy drinking. Also, the 26 percent rise in per capita consumption in the United States between 1961 and 1971 coincided with an increase in the death rate due to cirrhosis from 11.3 to 15.4 per 100,000 people. This rate would be an estimated 3 to 4 per 100,000 people if no alcohol were consumed.

Prohibition offers another example of how increases in price, reductions in consumption, and improvements in public health are linked. Statistics from this period uniformly indicate that drinking declined markedly as a result of Prohibition, especially among blue-collar workers. At the same time, deaths from cirrhosis and alcohol overdoses dropped to their lowest levels ever in the twentieth century. During the first years of Prohibition arrests for public drunkenness and admissions to mental hospitals for alcoholic psychoses (delirium tremens and dementias) plunged.

Some direct tests of the relations between the tax rates on alcohol, its consumption, and the effects of alcohol abuse have been performed by Philip Cook and his colleagues at Duke University. Cook examined the effects of 39 different increases in state liquor taxes between 1961 and 1975. These increases ranged from 4 cents to 28 cents on a fifth of 80 proof liquor (the federal tax during this time stayed constant at $1.68). He found not only a direct link between these price increases and consumption but also a connection between these price increases and two of the most serious consequences of alcohol use—cirrhosis of the liver and highway fatalities.

Whenever a state increased its liquor tax, Cook compared the change in that state's per capita consumption of alcohol with the changes in per capita consumption for all other states during that year. If the price of alcohol had an effect on consumption, the state in which the tax increased would be likely to have a relatively negative change in consumption. In 30 out of 39 cases, Cook found this to be true. "This is very strong evidence that an increase in tax reduces reported liquor sales in a state," he concluded.

Cook next applied this analysis to the death rates from cirrhosis for each of the states. Cirrhosis is a disease that generally develops after many years of heavy drinking. But because it is to some extent an interruptible disease, a decline in drinking could have an immediate effect on cirrhosis mortality. At any given time there is a reservoir of people who are within one year of dying from cirrhosis. If some of these people reduce their drinking because of a tax increase, the progress of their disease will slow and the rate of death from cirrhosis will go down.

Cook found that states with increased liquor taxes tended to have decreased cirrhosis mortality, a statistical result that could happen by chance just one time in fourteen. He concluded, "There is considerable statistical evidence that a liquor tax increase causes an immediate and substantial reduction in cirrhosis mortality." Cook also applied this analysis to the rate of highway fatalities in each state. Again, he found that mortality was linked to changes in the price of alcohol, an outcome that could result by chance just 4 percent of the time.

A more recent study by Cook and George Tauchen further quantified the link between tax increases and cirrhosis mortality.[2] Based on 1981 prices, their study found that an increase in the federal liquor tax of 16 cents on a fifth of 80 proof spirits would reduce the nation's cirrhosis mortality rate by 1.9 percent. This effect "is far from trivial," Cook says. "According to this estimate, a doubling of the U.S. federal liquor tax would reduce the nation's cirrhosis mortality rate by a figure in the neighborhood of 20 percent."

Other researchers have found the magnitude of this potential reduction striking. "The effect estimated by Cook and Tauchen

---

[2]P. J. Cook and G. Tauchen. The effect of liquor taxes on heavy drinking. *Bell Journal of Economics* 13 (1982):379-390.

is extraordinarily large," says Jeffrey Harris of the Massachusetts Institute of Technology. "A 20 percent decline would mean a postponement of about 6,000 deaths annually." Harris cautions, however, that "several additional lines of research are needed to fill in the gaps in the taxation-cirrhosis story." Among these are the response of individuals to price increases in alcohol, the shifts in demand among liquor, wine, and beer as the price of each changes, and the prevalence trend of cirrhosis that is not related to drinking.

More recent studies have begun to fill some of these gaps, and support for the linkage between alcohol price increases and cirrhosis mortality is increasing, though some students of alcohol issues remain dubious about effects of the size Cook and Tauchen estimate. Balancing such doubts against the results of systematic analyses, the National Research Council panel on alcohol abuse found the evidence sufficiently strong to conclude: "Alcohol consumption and the problems caused by it respond to the price of alcoholic beverages, and we infer that the large reductions in the real cost of alcohol to consumers in recent years are likely to have exacerbated drinking problems. . . . Therefore we see good grounds for incorporating an interest in the prevention of alcohol problems into the setting of tax rates on alcohol."

Options for Increasing Alcohol Taxes

If the federal government decided to raise taxes on alcohol, it could do so in many different ways. One option would be to restore the federal tax in real terms to its 1951 level. This would raise the federal taxes on distilled liquors from $1.92 for a fifth of 80 proof liquor to about $5.00. Federal taxes on beer would rise to about 50 cents on a six-pack and to as much as $2.00 on a 750-milliliter bottle of fortified wine.

A less extreme but still substantial step would be for the federal government to double its taxes on alcohol, as it did for cigarettes in 1982. A six-pack of beer would cost 16 cents more, all other things being equal. A fifth of 80 proof liquor would cost nearly $2.00 more. Overall, if the tax increase were fully passed on to consumers, the price of liquor would go up by about 24 percent.

The amount of revenue this would generate for the government would depend on how people responded to the higher prices. If people bought just as much liquor as they do now and simply paid the higher prices, federal revenues would double, going from around $5.5 billion to $12 billion. If people drank less but spent just as much money as they do now, a greater portion of their expenditures would go for taxes and federal revenues would rise from $5.5 billion to $10 billion. Similarly, if the federal government returned its taxes to the 1951 level in real terms and people spent no more money on alcohol than they do now, federal revenues from alcohol taxes would rise to $15 billion.

These hypothetical tax increases are given only as examples, not as concrete proposals. As discussed later in this chapter, real tax increases would be much more complex, as would be the responses to those increases. One of these complications is that it may make sense to change taxes on different kinds of alcohol by different amounts. Under the current system distilled spirits are taxed much more heavily than beer and table wine. Per ounce of pure alcohol, liquor is taxed at 19 cents, beer at 6 cents, and table wine at about 1 cent. In part, this reflects the continued sway of the temperance idea that beer and wine are drinks of moderation and less harmful than distilled spirits.

Research has cast doubt on the validity of this preconception. Drunk drivers and alcoholics report drinking beer and wine as well as hard liquor. The major diseases associated with drinking depend only on the consumption of alcohol, not on the type of beverage in which it comes.

It may therefore be more appropriate to tax alcoholic beverages according to their alcohol content. For instance, if the federal taxes on beer and wine were made equal to the tax on liquor in these terms, a six-pack of beer would cost 35 cents more and an average size bottle of wine would cost about 50 cents more. Such a tax increase would raise more revenues for the federal government than would simply doubling the tax rates on all three beverage types.

Complexities of Increasing Alcohol Taxes

There are several adverse consequences of raising alcohol taxes, and these, too, must be considered in establishing policies. One frequently heard objection is that alcohol taxes are indiscriminate, that they affect the drinker who is unlikely to have any problems with alcohol as well as the drinker who is. As noted in Chapter 2, however, it is often difficult to make this distinction. Also, higher taxes on alcohol may have benefits that apply to everyone in society. If they succeed in reducing the number of problems associated with alcohol, everyone would profit from safer highways, lower automobile and health insurance premiums, and fewer problems among friends and acquaintances.

Another question about higher alcohol taxes is whether they would overburden America's heaviest drinkers. Because just 5 percent of all adults drink 50 percent of the alcohol consumed in the United States, this small part of the population would pay about half of the increased taxes on alcohol. If some portion of these people are physiologically addicted to alcohol, might they drink just as much and pay the extra cost, making their lives more difficult without affecting their dependence on alcohol?

The work of Philip Cook and other researchers points in a different direction. Because people who contract cirrhosis are generally very heavy drinkers, cirrhosis death rates are a commonly used proxy measure of alcoholism. Thus a drop in cirrhosis death rates with an increase in the price of alcohol, which is the correlation Cook demonstrated, is evidence that very heavy drinkers are changing their consumption in response to price. Other researchers have used related measures to show that the drinking habits of alcoholics and other problem drinkers are not immune to the laws of supply and demand.

Another point that should be made is that people who drink excessively suffer proportionately more of the physical, social, economic, and emotional problems associated with drinking. In this sense, an increased tax on alcohol is more selective than it might appear. If excessive drinkers reduce their consumption in response to a higher tax, they could suffer fewer health problems and be more successful at their jobs. Thus their financial situation could improve because of a tax increase, although as usual this would vary from person to person.

Excessive drinkers also tend to use more of the public services provided for alcohol-related problems. These drinkers place expensive demands on medical care, alcoholism treatment, minimum income maintenance, and other social services. Tax receipts from alcohol sales already cover some of the public outlays for the portions of these services that go for alcohol problems. But, as we will see in the last section of this chapter, policymakers may wish to make this link explicit by requiring that increased taxes help pay for more extensive services.

One last question to be considered is how much more heavily higher alcohol taxes fall on poor families than on wealthier ones. In principle, excise taxes on alcohol are regressive in that they equal a lower percentage of a household's income as that income goes up. However, they are not as regressive in practice. Surveys show that purchases of alcohol increase as incomes rise, implying that wealthier people would also pay more of a tax increase. The consumption of alcohol "markedly increases with income," says Jeffrey Harris. "As in the case of tobacco, the reduced consumption at very low incomes reflects to some degree a large number of older, low-income abstainers." Even when age is taken into account, however, alcohol use increases with income.

Limits on the Availability of Alcohol

The price of alcohol is only one of many factors that influence how much, where, and when people drink. Other important factors are those that influence how easy it is to get alcohol. Over the last three decades legal restrictions on the availability of alcohol have generally eased. Minimum drinking ages have gone down (though recently they have been going back up), alcohol has been sold at more kinds of places, and these places have kept longer hours. It seems clear that if alcoholic beverages are sold in more restaurants, cafeterias, sports arenas, theaters, and other places, consumption will rise.

Federal, state, and local governments regulate these sales in various ways. They set minimum drinking ages. They control the number, location, and kinds of retail outlets. And they control the operation of these outlets by specifying legal hours of sale, setting minimum or maximum purchases per customer, requiring that food be served with drinks, prohibiting sales to drunk customers, requiring that operators maintain orderly premises, and so on.

Using this apparatus of regulation to prevent alcohol-related problems need not entail a return to the severe restrictions of the past. Less drastic changes can also influence the amount or the setting in which people drink. For instance, asks Robert Reynolds of San Diego County's Department of Health Services, "Is there any real reason to continue the sale of beer and wine in a stadium after the seventh inning, when people are about to drive out? Or in recreation sites? . . . These are areas of availability that do not specifically have to do with licensing regulations, but with local values and mores."

Regulations on availability can also be used in more traditional ways, especially to counter specific local problems. "There are many strategies that are the prerogatives of local governments, such as zoning, that can be used in heavily impacted areas," says Reynolds. "Why should a community not choose to refuse more outlets if, for example, its alcohol-related crime rate is already 20 percent above the norm? Communities can mobilize around those kinds of issues and have an impact on the number of outlets permitted."

The results of broad changes in the availability of alcohol are sometimes difficult to predict. For guidance, researchers have often looked to the experience of other countries, such as Finland in the 1960s and 1970s. There a long period of liberalization during the 1960s culminated in the passage of the Alcohol Act of 1969. This act abolished restrictions that had banned alcohol sales in rural areas, lowered the drinking age for certain beverages, and permitted retail shops to sell beer with a higher alcohol content.

According to Dan Beauchamp, who has studied this episode intensively, "The effects of these changes took virtually everyone by surprise." During the first year after the act, per capita

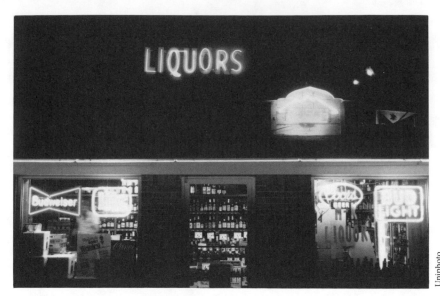

Uniphoto

Outlets selling alcohol have multiplied in recent years, making alcohol available at a much wider range of places and times.

consumption rose 46 percent. By 1975 the Finns were drinking 156 percent more beer, 96 percent more spirits, and 87 percent more wine. Total per capita consumption was more than twice what it had been just seven years before.

The Alcohol Act of 1969 was not the only catalyst for increased drinking during those years. Consumer expenditures per capita were also increasing, and general cultural attitudes were becoming more liberal, especially among young people. But the act contributed to the creation of a dense distribution network in Finland that had the effect of increasing consumption.

Does this experience have any relevance for the United States, where a dense distribution network for the most part already exists? Research on variations in the number or location of outlets in various parts of the United States has been inconclusive, and there are specific situations about which little is known. For instance, do sales of alcoholic beverages in groceries or drugstores increase the amount consumed? Do minimarts attached to gas stations lead to more drunk driving?

Overall, concludes Michael Goodstadt of the Alcoholism and Drug Addiction Research Foundation in Toronto, the issue of availability is much like that of violence on television. The data suggesting a link between greater availability and more drinking are not conclusive. But they are strong enough for policymakers to view with caution any action that would make alcohol more available. "Quite a number of studies, in addition to common sense, would suggest that we stop making alcohol ever more available," says Goodstadt. "The data are not sterling, you would not stake your entire reputation on any single study, but collectively you would say: 'Hold on.' "

Political Realities

Legislators must take into account many competing concerns besides public health in making decisions about alcohol policy. For instance, when Congress raised the federal tax on cigarettes from 8 cents to 16 cents per pack in 1982 (it too had not been changed since the 1950s), the incidence of lung cancer may not have been as forceful an argument as the need to help reduce a skyrocketing federal deficit. Still, if people smoke less as a result of the price hike, one effect of the tax increase will be an improvement in health.

Increasing the taxes on alcohol could have this same dual effect. "Taxation has the clear advantage of working at a distance from people and accomplishing more than one end, which in politics is always good," says Dan Beauchamp. Whatever a legislator's motivation, higher taxes on alcohol could both reduce alcohol problems and raise public revenues. "There are a number of alternatives for reducing the U.S. budget deficit," says Cook. "Few of them have the substantial beneficial side effects that would result from raising the alcohol excise tax rates."

Then again, there are a number of powerful factors working against an increase in alcohol taxes. For instance, higher taxes at the federal or state level may affect the net receipts of the alcoholic beverage industry and impinge on the profit margins or business practices of brewers, vintners, distillers, and the thousands of restaurants, taverns, liquor stores, and other outlets that sell alcohol. These effects will be closely scrutinized, for, as John Vassallo of New Jersey's Division of Alcoholic Beverage Control points out, "Alcoholic beverage taxes or profits (in the control states) are very important to the economy of almost every state."

People who suspect they would be adversely affected by a tax increase can be expected to make their voices heard in a legislature. The alcoholic beverage industry has traditionally been a powerful constituency, and their influence on alcohol policy can be strong. Michael Fox of the Ohio General Assembly has experienced this kind of pressure firsthand:

> A lot of folks make a good living selling alcoholic beverages, and they have for years contended that tax policy affects consumption. I spent four years on the state government committee in Ohio, and all we heard in that committee were what we affectionately called "booze bills." One after another, the tavern owners and the wholesalers would come before us and say, "You are putting us out of business, this is affecting our sales. . . ."

> I mention this as a word of caution. There is a real world out there in which legislators get beat over the head. If a bill goes to a state government committee or a similar committee in one of the legislatures, it will have a hard time getting out of committee because such committees are dominated by people who are generally friendly to the industry.

One way that legislators have made tax increases more acceptable to the public is by earmarking portions of the revenues obtained for use in specific alcohol treatment or prevention programs. Small taxes on alcohol can generate relatively large revenues for alcohol programs, and several states have already taken steps in this direction. New York State requires that half of the money collected from drunk driving fines be returned to the county where the arrest was made for education and prevention programs. Other states require drunk drivers to pay for their own treatment programs. Such links between cause and effect can be politically essential. "It has become very clear," says Alfred McAlister of the University of Texas, "that the political acceptability of such a tax increase depends on whether the public perceives some connection, an earmarking or diversion of a portion of the funds, to prevention programs."

But the earmarking of funds also has its difficulties. According to Jane Smith Patterson, Secretary of Administration for the State of North Carolina, state legislatures have traditionally resisted such proposals. "At the state level, legislatures and governors across the country flatly dislike the earmarking of public revenues and will fight you even though they agree with what you want to do. They do not want funds to be dedicated in the actual excise tax act. They want the funds raised first."

If revenues are not earmarked, there is always the possibility that other demands—possibly even other health care needs—will siphon them off from programs to prevent alcohol problems. To this problem Patterson answers, "You will just have to sell your state legislature on prevention."

5

What Servers Can Do

*I*N OVER HALF THE STATES in the nation, commercial servers of alcoholic beverages can be held liable for damage or injuries caused by their drunken or underage patrons. These servers can include bartenders, waiters and waitresses, the managers or operators of an establishment that sells alcohol, or the owners of an establishment. In some states this liability extends even to noncommercial servers, such as hosts at a party or bartenders at an informal social gathering.

These dramshop laws, as they are known, establish civil liabilities. They complement both a state's Alcoholic Beverage Control (ABC) laws and its criminal sanctions against such acts as selling alcohol to a minor. Courts around the country have repeatedly upheld the validity of these laws. "Such business responsibilities are common to other professions offering services to the public," says James Mosher of the Medical Research Institute of San Francisco. "The primary debate should not be the existence of that responsibility but rather its scope."

Despite their solid legal standing, dramshop laws have been difficult to apply. A commercial server can be held liable only if he or she sold alcohol to an underage or "obviously intoxicated" person. The vague wording of the latter prohibition offers little guidance either to a server or to members of a jury. Noncommercial servers, such as social hosts, fraternity bartenders, or employers, have only been held liable for serving underage drinkers. When court cases in Iowa and California implied that social hosts could be held liable for serving obviously intoxicated guests, each state quickly passed legislation contravening the decision.

This chapter concentrates on commercial rather than noncommercial servers for several reasons. For one thing, experience with dramshop laws is still limited. At this early stage, commercial establishments offer the best setting for learning about effective ways for servers to protect their patrons and guests.

Also, people who have been drinking in public establishments tend to make up a large fraction of drunk drivers. In one roadside survey, 44 percent of the drivers with blood alcohol contents above 0.10 percent were driving to, from, or between public eating and drinking places.

Finally, changes made in commercial establishments cannot help but carry over into private life. "Serving practices in private settings will inevitably be affected both by the public example of concern set by new professional practices and by the diffusion of experience gained by employees, trainers, and researchers into the common body of knowledge and custom," says Mosher.

Bartender Training

The most obvious way for a drinking establishment to avoid dramshop liability is for its servers to see that patrons do not get drunk or do not harm themselves or others if they do. Servers have several such ways to intervene on behalf of their customers. They can make it less convenient or acceptable for a person to get drunk or try to drive while drunk. They can suggest that a person wait to sober up or arrange for a friend or taxi to take that person home. They can even physically restrain a person or report to the police someone who insists on driving drunk. As might be expected, none of these options is easy. To a bar or tavern owner, intervention can mean lower profits. To a commercial server, intervention can mean the inconvenience of arranging a ride or a place to stay or the sheer unpleasantness of telling a person that he or she is incompetent to drive. In many cases, servers need special training to be able to carry out these tasks successfully.

This is one of the reasons for the several "server intervention" programs that have sprung up across the country in recent years. Typically, these programs offer training sessions on the effects of alcohol on the body, signs of intoxication, the legal responsibilities of servers, ways to cut off service to people who are drinking too much, how to handle intoxicated people, management practices that support server intervention, and the nature of alcoholism and its treatment. These courses have attracted considerable attention from individuals and groups concerned with drinking and its harmful consequences. The Presidential Task Force on Drunk Driving, Mothers Against Drunk Driving (MADD), the National Highway Traffic Safety Administration, and several state task forces on drunk driving have all recommended that aspects of these programs be instituted more widely.

One of the most comprehensive and well studied of these programs was conducted by the California ABC Department from 1977 to 1980. At the beginning of the program, people arrested for drunk driving were asked where they had had their last drink. When a certain drinking establishment was listed three or more times, the ABC Department contacted the establishment and offered a server training program. Participation was voluntary, and at first many licensees were suspicious. But most did participate. By the end of the first year, during which over 5,000 servers were trained, more requests were coming in for training than the department could handle.

The city of Madison, Wisconsin, took a different approach to ensuring that servers receive training in intervention techniques. In 1981 it passed a law requiring that all commercial servers of alcoholic beverages take an alcohol awareness training program before obtaining a license. The program set up to meet this requirement covers four main topics: city and state laws, the effects of alcohol and other drugs, alcoholism and alcoholism treatment, and human relations and marketing. Local police, alcohol-related programs, and tavern associations have all supported the effort.

Another innovative server intervention program has arisen in Amherst, Massachusetts. There James Peters has used both legal means and voluntary cooperation to reduce the number of happy hours, institute citywide server training sessions, control advertising, and encourage the cutting off of intoxicated patrons. Largely because of his efforts, legislation has been introduced at the state level to require training as a condition of licensing.

Other server intervention programs have also been established in the past few years. The University of Minnesota has developed a community-based program in which licensees are encouraged to sponsor training sessions for their employees. The New York State Division of Alcoholism and Alcohol Abuse, in cooperation with the New York State Restaurant Association, has conducted seminars for commercial servers. MADD in California and the Health Education Foundation in Washington, D.C., have also set up seminar series. "These programs represent a significant step in server intervention policy," concludes Mosher. "They are practical efforts to incorporate commercial alcohol establishments into a prevention effort."

Making Server Intervention More Effective

Bartender training programs are a valuable step forward, but they are only one component of what could be a comprehensive approach to server intervention. As with all prevention efforts, the pursuit of a number of different strategies simultaneously can have the greatest effect with the least restraint on personal freedoms. In the area of server intervention, there are several areas into which current programs could profitably expand, including the drinking environment, management training, and legal support.

With regard to the drinking environment, several key questions arise. What are the interior and exterior designs of a drinking place? Where is the alcohol being served? And what kinds of transportation facilities, either public or private, are available for patrons?

The design of a drinking establishment can help or hinder a responsible server. For instance, many bartender training pro-

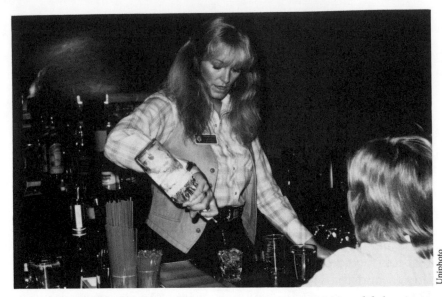

Uniphoto

Bartenders are often particularly well situated to observe the drinking of their patrons and to intervene when necessary.

grams emphasize that servers should make frequent, unobstrusive observations of their patrons. Yet this may be impossible in bars, taverns, or restaurants with certain physical layouts, such as large, impersonal lounges or dance halls.

The design and characteristics of a drinking establishment can also influence how often intervention is necessary. Studies have shown that physical and social settings have an effect on how much a person drinks. Drinkers take cues from the people around them about how much and how fast they should drink. Sometimes these influences moderate drinking, as is often the case when one drinks at home in the company of family. At other times these influences increase drinking, as can happen when one is out on the town with friends.

By taking account of these less tangible influences on drinking, servers can both lessen the need for intervention and make intervention easier if the need does arise. According to Mosher, "Such variables as crowdedness, noise, availability of nonalcoholic beverages and food and of nondrinking activities that promote sociability may substantially reduce the need for interventions by bartenders and other employees."

Another important environmental factor involves the establishment's location. If a patron becomes inebriated, he or she needs some way other than driving a private automobile to get home. Some locales have recently begun offering free taxi, minibus, or public transportation services during peak drinking periods, like holiday weekends. Such efforts could be made more often, especially for popular drinking spots or on special drinking occasions. Alcohol outlets should at least have a way of calling taxis for drunk patrons, and taxis must arrive quickly if they are to be of much use.

Many of these changes in the drinking environment require that managers be committed to intervention, a factor that past training programs have sometimes overlooked. "There is a tendency to focus merely on the front line—bartenders, cocktail waitresses, and other employees actually in contact with the establishment's customers," says Mosher. "An effective intervention program, however, may require a number of reforms in management practices, including such variables as the number of employees on the job, the number of patrons allowed on the premises, the interior design, the commitment to alternative forms of transportation, the hours of operation, the use of promotional techniques, etc."

Finally, past server intervention programs have made little use of legal support. An exception to this rule is the program in Madison, Wisconsin, which made training a prerequisite of licensing. Other jurisdictions, whether at the state or local level, could pass similar laws to guarantee that every server of alcoholic beverages receives some measure of training.

The other legal incentive for server intervention programs is the dramshop laws themselves. As mentioned, these laws have usually proven to be too vague to persuade servers to change their policies. Moreover, insurance companies have often shortcut the intent of the laws by settling out of court on unjustified claims. This can make the owner of a drinking establishment reluctant to change house policies, since such changes do little to protect against unjustified claims. Also, since establishments often buy insurance to cover their liability, settlements help transform dramshop laws into what Mosher calls "imperfect victim-compensation mechanisms."

Interest has recently been building in ways to change these laws to make them more effective. Some of this interest comes from the servers themselves, who are being squeezed by the high premiums charged for liability insurance (in California these premiums went up 500 to 1,000 percent in the wake of certain court cases that went against commercial servers). One such change would involve broadening dramshop laws to include an assessment of the server's overall level of responsibility. The liability of a server would then depend on whether the server had taken reasonable steps to protect other people from harm. "For example," says Mosher, "a server who institutes a training program for employees, implements management practices that encourage compliance, and is attentive to environmental variables such as alternative transportation for intoxicated patrons could be protected as a matter of law from dramshop suits, assuming he or she can prove that the procedures were followed on a given occasion." Such changes in the dramshop laws would be a strong inducement for participation in server intervention programs, especially if insurance companies acknowledged that participation with lower liability insurance rates.

Options for Businesses

Many drinking establishments and other businesses around the country have supported server intervention programs, and some have made prominent commitments to intervention techniques. An example is the S & A Restaurant Corporation, which owns about 300 restaurants nationwide. The corporation has instituted a wide-ranging server intervention program. The key to the program, according to the corporation's vice-president and general counsel Roger Thomson, is the sharing of responsibility between the restaurant and its patrons:

We are spending a great deal of time, money, and effort to educate our employees *and* our patrons on the sharing of responsibility. . . .

Nationwide, we have posted notices in some of our restaurants to remind our customers that they have a responsibility, and we will refuse to serve

WHAT SERVERS CAN DO / 69

them if we think they are not taking this responsibility. We also have blood alcohol content charts posted in some restrooms and telephone booths. If we think that somebody may be drinking too much, we may serve them protein- and fat-rich foods that absorb alcohol more quickly. We may also place in our new menus a nonalcoholic beverage section that receives top billing. We have game areas that allow people to feel that they do not have to sit and drink first to enjoy a meal, and we are initiating other diversions for people who choose not to drink alcohol. Where we have been able to strike deals with taxi companies, our restaurants have a hot line to the taxi company: Just pick up the phone, which is a direct line, and we pay for the cab to take home a patron who has had too much to drink.

To educate our staff, we invite the local police and the local alcohol councils to speak to our employees frequently. In our newspaper, which goes to all our restaurants, there is often an article on some aspect of alcohol. We help our employees recognize the signs of intoxication and we give them support to cut an intoxicated person off. On the community level, we funnel money into various school systems to produce posters on responsibility and alcohol. We work with Mothers Against Drunk Driving and other groups on various local issues. We are trying to be responsible.

Programs such as that of the S & A Restaurant Corporation are an encouraging development, as is the widespread attention now being focused on this approach. At the same time, much more needs to be done before it will be possible to institute server intervention programs widely. Many different groups and organizations—including ABC boards, insurance commissions, law enforcement agencies, citizen groups, researchers, educators, and legislators—will have to coordinate their actions to make these programs a success. According to Mosher, the federal government must take a special part in this interplay of initiatives. "The federal government," he says, "through the National Institute on Alcohol Abuse and Alcoholism, needs to take the lead in this process, providing financial resources for the necessary research and evaluation studies, offering technical assistance to interested groups, acting as an information clearinghouse, and ensuring that duplication of effort is minimized."

6

Drinking by Young People

"*A*DOLESCENCE is a very special time. We cannot treat teenagers as little children, using naive prevention strategies. We cannot treat them as adults because they are in a vulnerable period of internal stress, confusion, and irrationality. They are particularly vulnerable because of their tendency to be more loyal to their friends than to their own welfare." M. "Keith" Schuchard of the Parental Resource Institute for Drug Education in Atlanta has put her finger on a central problem of attempts to prevent alcohol abuse among young people. Adolescents are making their way through a particularly fast-moving and transitional part of their lives. Most are beginning a process that will eventually lead to their moving away from their parents. Yet most adolescents are not yet ready to make *all* their own decisions, to establish an independent life free of parental constraints.

The conflicts of this gradual separation exacerbate what is already a difficult time. Almost all adolescents suffer from a great deal of insecurity. They worry about their bodies, their likability, the opinions of their friends, their family relationships. Adolescents have many problems to work out. Some they will successfully resolve, some they will forget, and some will follow them into adulthood.

Adolescence is also the time when many people face their first inducements to drink. (The use of the term adolescent should not disguise the fact that at least some people start drinking earlier than adolescence, when they are really still children.) Laws against selling alcohol to people under a certain age do reduce the amount that adolescents drink. But these laws fall far short of imposing absolute abstinence on this group. According to national surveys, 80 percent of high school seniors have had their first drink before they turn 18—the lowest minimum drinking age in the country. Over one-third of all high school students, including half of all 16- to 17-year-olds, report drinking within the past 30 days.

The question of why adolescents drink may be even more difficult to answer than the question of why adults drink. Clearly, peer pressure plays a large role in the initiation of drinking. But there are many other factors that also contribute, from family situations to availability to the intangible influence of an individual's personality. At least some of these factors can be influenced very little by prevention programs, no matter how skillfully such programs may be designed.

Adolescents are also under particularly intense pressure from the mass media and popular culture. During a stage in their lives when they are particularly susceptible to such messages, adolescents are barraged by enticements to drink in television shows and advertising. Alcohol is a theme in popular music, in comic strips, and particularly in movies. (Who cannot remember a popular film in which the protagonist was an incorrigible, but ultimately attractive, drunk?) Schuchard particularly objects to such messages on young people's T-shirts as "Party till you puke," "Avoid hangovers, stay drunk," and "I don't have a drinking problem—I drink, I get drunk, I fall down. No problem."

This blitz of promotion, says Schuchard, continually antagonizes parents and educators who are trying to teach young people about drinking. "The industry talks about responsible marketing," she says, "but I see alcoholic milk shakes in stores and I hear advertising on teen-oriented radio stations for beer, wine, and other kinds of drinks. . . . There are mixed-up, muddy messages going to the adolescent, who is supposed to become adult and responsible in handling intoxicating chemicals that basically make him or her irresponsible."

Does the Drinking Age Make a Difference?

Every state in the nation has a minimum drinking age, ranging from 18 to 21. As of June 1, 1985, 3 states set the minimum age at 18, 12 set the limit at 19, 2 set the limit at 20, and 34 (including the District of Columbia) set the limit at 21 (although several of these allowed beer sales to 18- or 19-year-olds).

The primary justification for drinking ages greater than 18 is concern over traffic accidents involving young people who have been drinking. Each year approximately 5,000 lives are lost in alcohol-related traffic accidents in which the driver is under 21. According to the National Highway Traffic Safety Administra-

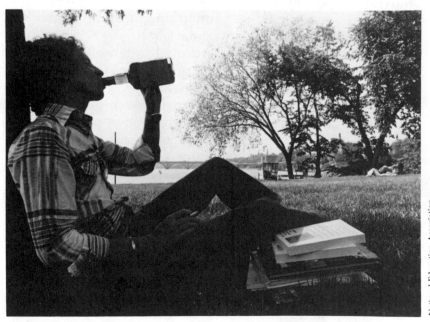

National Education Association

Alcohol abuse can be a major problem on college campuses, where most students reach the minimum drinking age in an environment marked by ready access to alcohol and great personal freedom.

tion (NHTSA), 20 percent of all fatal highway accidents involve drivers under 21, although this group makes up less than 10 percent of the total number of licensed drivers. For people aged 15 to 34, automobile accidents are the single greatest cause of death.

The bare statistics about young people, drinking, and accidental deaths do little to convey the depth of the tragedies that strike so many families each year. There are few events more shattering than the death or permanent disablement of a person on the threshold of a full, adult life. It is the emotional anguish of these families that has inspired such volunteer groups as Mothers Against Drunk Driving (MADD), Students Against Drunk Driving (SADD), and Remove Intoxicated Drivers (RID). Drawing on their own grief, these groups have inspired efforts by others to deal more effectively with the problem.

Between 1970 and 1973, 24 states reduced their minimum drinking ages. The rationale for making such changes was then and still is straightforward and reasonable. State and federal laws give 18-year-olds most of the rights and responsibilities associated with adulthood—among them the right to vote, seek many elective offices, enter into contractual agreements, and serve in the armed forces. It seems logically consistent to also confer the right to drink on this group.

In the wake of these reductions in the minimum drinking age, a number of studies sought to assess how these changes would affect highway fatality rates among the young. These studies did not automatically anticipate that this rate would be higher; there are factors that can *decrease* drinking-driving accidents among the young when the drinking age goes down. For instance, teenagers might be less likely to drink in their cars if bars and taverns are open to them, or they might stop driving to neighboring jurisdictions with lower minimum drinking ages. The studies generally found, however, that reductions in the drinking age did cause a small but consistent increase in the rate of crashes and deaths involving younger drivers.

Based on such findings, NHTSA and many private organizations have concluded that, despite the logical consistency of an 18-year drinking age, it is better to set drinking ages at 21 and consign fewer young people to die each year on the highways. NHTSA itself recommended to all of the states that they raise their minimum drinking ages to 21. According to NHTSA's Barry Sweedler, this recommendation received support "from across the board." In addition, a Gallup poll has shown that 77 percent of the population supports legislation that would raise the drinking age to 21. Surprisingly enough, even among 18- to 20-year-olds 58 percent support such legislation.

In 1984 Congress passed a law that would reduce federal highway funds to states that have not raised their drinking ages to 21 by 1986. This is a strong incentive for states with minimum ages below 21 to raise them. But it remains the states' prerogative to set the minimum drinking age, and influential constituencies within states have a stake in keeping the drinking age low. "Where a proposal to raise the drinking age has been voted on by a legislative body in this country, it has not lost," says Sweedler. "But in many states it has been bottled up in committee, primarily because of strong lobbying efforts by people who sell alcohol primarily to youth."

What Can Schools Do?

Another focus of attempts to shape drinking habits is the schools. This emphasis is definitely not new. Schools have been teaching students about drinking since the nineteenth century. Originally a product of the temperance movement, this education was for many years strongly antialcohol. Lessons painted a grim picture of alcohol's disastrous effects on character, family life, and the fabric of society. Ruin was predicted for the vast majority of people who drank at all.

With the beginning of the alcoholism movement in the 1930s and 1940s, alcohol education became more health-oriented and factual. In the years that followed it grew progressively less colorful and less extensive. By the 1960s, alcohol education had shifted its focus primarily to alcoholism. Avoiding alarmist interpretations, it presented alcoholism as a disease to which every drinker had a small but real risk of succumbing.

In the 1970s attention to alcohol education increased markedly. At the beginning of the decade the National Institute on Alcohol Abuse and Alcoholism was founded. The NIAAA in turn set up the National Center for Alcohol Education and the National Clearinghouse for Alcohol Information, in part as sources of new educational materials. The increasing problem of drug use in the schools also strengthened alcohol education, as drug programs in general were expanded. Finally, teenage drinking came to be seen as a modern, worsening problem, although in fact research shows that drinking among teenagers has changed relatively little over the past 20 years.

Despite this new attention to alcohol education, the effectiveness of these programs remains open to doubt. Much of today's alcohol education seeks to produce lifelong changes in a person's drinking. In effect, the goal of this education is to "inoculate" a person against future drinking problems. This goal seems unrealistic for several reasons. In the first place, drinking practices tend to change dramatically over a person's lifetime. Information absorbed about alcohol in school is not likely to have much direct effect on behavior many years later. Also, many attitudes toward drinking are learned outside school. Students pay little attention when teachers start discussing issues of lifestyle patterns that were learned at home or elsewhere outside the classroom. As the National Research Council panel on alcohol abuse concludes, ". . . [T]he ambitions of school-based alcohol education programs are too grand."

It may be more practical for schools to lower their sights. Students must cope with many problems related to alcohol while they are in school: violence, traffic accidents, diminished academic performance. These problems seem the logical subject of school-based educational programs. Rather than concentrating on lifelong drinking practices, programs could aim to achieve specific behavioral goals. Students could be taught that they are responsible for violent, reckless, or self-defeating behavior, whether they are drunk or sober. According to the panel, "High schools and universities should adopt the objective of shaping drinking practices for the student populations while they are of school age and should register success if they succeed in reducing drinking and problems associated with drinking for their current populations. This reorientation may not require much change in current approaches and materials, but it would certainly require replacing the prevailing vague objectives of school-based alcohol education programs with clear behavioral goals."

One program that draws on these principles, known as the Shalom program, was founded in the Philadelphia schools by Sister Madeleine Boyd. It is staffed by professional social workers, psychologists, and guidance counselors. In sessions during study periods and before and after school, the program lays out the possible consequences of drinking or drug use and discusses how students can avoid them. "It is a highly structured discussion group from which they can learn new skills and at the same time gain new knowledge, techniques, and strategies to implement this knowledge," says Boyd. "The facts are presented in various ways: through psychodrama, magazines, music, videotapes, and movies."

The Shalom program points toward an important component of any effort to influence drinking by the young. A number of studies have concluded that peer pressure is the major factor in the initiation of drinking, smoking, and drug use. To counter this pressure, several experimental programs have used peers to teach counterarguments against smoking or drinking. In one study in California, 16-year-olds led 12-year-olds in sessions designed to make it easier for them to resist inducements to smoke or drink. The researchers had only the students' own reports to evaluate the program's effect, but students did report significantly less smoking and drinking. Similar results were achieved in Boston in a program that used "opinion leaders" nominated by their peers to direct classroom discussion.

What Can Parents Do?

The question of what parents can do should perhaps begin with what they are legally bound to do. Parents are legally liable for the behavior of minors in their home and under their supervision, whether the minors are their own children or someone else's. "If the daughter is having a slumber party and the parents are upstairs watching television, the kids get drunk from bottles out of the liquor cabinet and one of them drives off and kills someone, it is the host parents' responsibility," says Keith Schuchard. "If they did not know it was going on, that is neglect in the supervision of minors."

Reminding people of this legal liability has heightened the responsibility of all parties involved. "This is a tremendous public message," says Schuchard. "Even the kids thought it made sense. . . . The point made the teenagers recognize their own responsibility not to get parents in trouble."

This legal liability shades gradually into the realm of parental and ethical responsibilities. As with the legal issues, at least part of the justification for these latter responsibilities is the health of the child. "Parents are responsible for their children's health and make the rules about vaccinations, measles, and everything else medical; they should make it about drugs and alcohol," Schuchard says.

Health is also a relatively neutral subject on which parents can approach their children about alcohol. Adolescents are very concerned about their body images and about the changes their bodies are undergoing. Parents can take advantage of this concern by telling their children about the potential consequences to health of drinking. To help make this possible, researchers should learn as much as possible about the physiological effects of alcohol and other drugs on young people.

Another way for parents to convey their attitudes about drinking to their children is by forming their own peer groups or networks, according to Schuchard. Within these networks, parents can form codes of behavior that apply to all of the children in the group. "Such a code does not have to cover everything, but it should cover illegal activity, the use of drugs and alcohol, getting into dangerous situations with automobiles, etc.," Schuchard says.

Parents in the network can watch over each other's children; for example, the children of working parents can check in with other parents after school. It is an idea based on a fundamental human value, a value that lies at the heart of a parent's concern over drinking by young people. "The parental instinct to protect a child's physical well-being is the strongest instinct in nature and in society," Schuchard says. "If we can tap that instinct and reinforce it with community support and legal sanctions, we *can* build an effective prevention movement."

Prevention at the College Level

When teenagers go away to college, the situation changes. For many of them it is the first time they have lived away from home. Parental oversight diminishes, the range of opportunity increases, the world can seem a much larger and freer place. For some students this is a dangerous combination.

Many students, faculty, administrators, and community members associated with universities have expressed concern over the amount and consequences of the drinking that goes on in college. One university that sought to channel that concern in constructive directions is the University of Massachusetts at Amherst. For 10 years beginning in 1973, this campus of 22,000 students, over half of whom live in university housing, was the site of a comprehensive program to prevent alcohol-related problems among its students, the Demonstration Alcohol Education Project (DAEP).

Problems associated with drinking were widespread on campus during DAEP. Over the years 1975-80, an average of 29 percent of students surveyed reported driving while intoxicated, 23 percent reported academic problems related to drinking, 17 percent reported minor physical problems associated with drinking, 16 percent reported alcohol-related abusive behavior, and 14 percent had trouble with their jobs because of alcohol. Smaller percentages reported property damage caused by drunkenness or dependence on alcohol.

DAEP sought to reduce these problems using posters, newspaper advertisements and articles, radio advertisements and interviews, and special displays in the student center. Each year about 10 percent of the students in the university also received intensive face-to-face instruction about drinking. Generally, these sessions involved small groups of students taught by other, trained students and were held in dormitories or classrooms. About half of 1 percent of all students participated in more than one discussion group or in formal courses dealing with alcohol. DAEP also trained about 5 percent of the university's staff and faculty each year, and it sought to study and modify various regulations involving alcohol.

Over the course of the program, several special projects were initiated that involved the broader university community as well as students. In many cases these projects evolved within the broader program as specific problems became apparent. "The needs often could not be adequately addressed until relevant individuals or groups in the community became sufficiently concerned to help effect necessary changes," says David Kraft of the university's Health Services Department.

One of these special projects was a comprehensive party-planning policy implemented in 1978 by a joint student-staff task force. This policy defined the responsibilities and training required of party planners, bartenders, security personnel, and staff supervisors for parties of different sizes.

In 1981 four young people who had been drinking were involved in a fatal accident in Amherst. This led to the Safety Action Program, a cooperative effort of the town and university. According to Kraft, this program "included both education about drinking and driving in the secondary schools and on college campuses, and stricter, highly visible enforcement of drunk driving laws with subsequent convictions."

In 1982 questions by off-campus bar owners about their liability for accidents led to an expansion of the on-campus bartender training to off-campus establishments. Also in 1982 a special educational effort called the Student Opportunity Program began working with students who had disciplinary problems related to alcohol.

DAEP was evaluated through an annual questionnaire, surveys of university staff members, archival data, and controlled studies of the educational efforts. These evaluations showed that most students did learn about alcohol problems and agreed about the need to control them. However, the questionnaires uncovered no significant decrease in either drinking or alcohol-related problems over the years of DAEP. Only among the students who were taught to train other students did alcohol problems significantly diminish. As in other programs of this type, it is possible to give people new knowledge without necessarily changing their behavior.

Despite the lack of a change in drinking practices, there were many indications of ways in which DAEP did have a positive effect. University faculty and staff recognized alcohol-related problems much earlier and acted to deal with them. Students were also more likely to confront their peers in an attempt to make them drink more safely. Specific environmental factors changed, such as more parties offering food and nonalcoholic beverages. When DAEP came to an end, many of its educational efforts were integrated into the ongoing activities of the groups that had been involved in the program.

According to Kraft, DAEP brought to the fore a number of observations that should be taken into account in designing similar programs. First of all, a university-based program should decide which alcohol-related problems concern university and community members the most. At the beginning of DAEP, campus and community leaders were most concerned about what seemed to be an increasing number of student alcoholics. But they soon saw the need to expand the program to include many other people. "Very quickly, key community members began to realize that the highest proportion of alcohol problems occurred among both regular and occasional heavy consumers of alcohol, only some of whom would be defined as 'alcoholic' by any standard criteria," says Kraft. "The focus of community alcohol program efforts rapidly shifted to preventing certain problems by a variety of strategies, only some of which focused on heavy drinkers, including alcoholics."

Once the problem is defined, programs like DAEP should enlist aid from as many groups and individuals as possible. Programs too often overlook such obvious partners as distribution centers (bars, restaurants, liquor stores, etc.), servers, police and medical personnel, and community leaders. These organizations and individuals may initially resist some of the changes a program seeks, but they can be valuable parts of a comprehensive approach to prevention.

Finally, programs like DAEP should be evaluated continuously and refined if necessary. "The evaluation methods used need not be highly advanced or complicated, but should be systematic and honest," says Kraft. "Systematic evaluation can also help ensure ongoing community funding and support even if efforts are only moderately successful."

In general, Kraft believes that community-based approaches to preventing alcohol problems work best by combining education with regulation. Neither alone is practical. To be effective, education alone would be too expensive, and regulation by itself can polarize community members around unpopular laws. But together they can complement each other by reinforcing and drawing attention to each other's messages. "A combination of education and regulation proved to be the most effective way to produce community-level changes at the University of Massachusetts," Kraft concludes.

7

Drinking and the Mass Media

IN 1980 A TEAM OF RESEARCHERS from Michigan State University carefully watched four episodes of television's top-rated prime-time fictional shows and eight episodes of the top-rated soap operas. Every time a character took a drink, the researchers made a note of it. Every time a character mentioned alcohol or acted drunk, the researchers made another entry in their logs. When they added up the number of times drinking was depicted, a remarkable statistic emerged.

"Television characters may not smoke or use drugs," observed Bradley Greenberg, head of the Michigan State study, "but they drink with prodigious frequency." In the prime-time shows, characters consumed alcoholic beverages an average of eight times every hour. In the top-rated soap operas, each hour averaged over two depictions of drinking.[1] People on television drink alcohol more often than they drink other beverages, the opposite of what happens in real life (see Figure 7-1). The bev-

---

[1]B. Greenberg. Television: Health issues on commercial television series. *Health Promotion and the Mass Media*. M. Trudeau and M. Angle, eds. Washington, D.C.: National Academy Press, 1981.

82

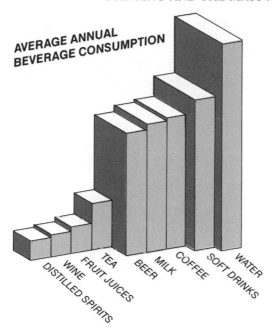

FIGURE 7.1   Americans drink far more nonalcoholic beverages than alcoholic beverages on the average, yet television shows generally portray alcohol as the most common beverage consumed. Of an average of 182.5 gallons drunk per year by all Americans, alcoholic beverages represent about 16 percent of the total and nonalcoholic beverages about 84 percent. Source: Alcohol Research Information Service.

erage consumed most often in television shows is distilled liquor, a substance that cannot be advertised on television because of industry self-regulation.

In the shows watched by the Michigan State researchers, virtually every depiction of drinking was positive. Drinking and drunkenness often tend to be presented in a humorous way on television. Sometimes drinking is shown as a way to solve problems, relieve tension, or blend in with a group. Drinking is generally a sophisticated, glamorous, mature act, a normal part of people's behavior. Rarely is it associated with any sort of problem, except in shows explicitly focused on alcohol problems. Characters in most shows seldom disapprove of another person's drinking, and when they do their disapproval tends to be mild.

Television is not the only mass medium through which people receive messages about drinking. But for many people it is the most important. Almost every home in America has at least one television set, and Americans spend an average of 30 hours a week watching television. When a person graduates from high school, he or she will probably have spent more time in front of a television than in a classroom. Throughout childhood and adolescence, television viewing takes up more hours on the average than any other single activity except sleeping.

As with violence on television, it is very difficult to prove that so much drinking on television leads to more drinking in real life. But the sheer quantity of drinking to which people are exposed on television is reason for concern. Given the amount of television young people watch and the number of drinking incidents portrayed, a person under the legal drinking age will watch an average of over 3,000 acts of drinking every year.

"Television has not been a very good educator about drinking in society," concludes Lawrence Wallack of the University of California at Berkeley. "The rate of drinking on television is greater than that in real life and the rate of problems associated with drinking tends to be much lower. . . . If indeed alcohol is a major public health problem and, as the panel estimates, is responsible for 50,000-75,000 deaths annually—you could not find this out from watching television."

Advertising Alcohol: A Billion-Dollar Business

Television and the other mass media deliver another important set of messages about drinking: advertisements for alcoholic beverages. Each year the alcoholic beverage industry spends over $1 billion advertising its products. "We will hear it on radio and see it on billboards, television, magazines, buses, subways, calendars, sports schedules, and most any other place where space is available," says Wallack. "The attention of the American public is clearly the focus of intense competition among alcoholic beverage producers."

It was not always this way. When Prohibition ended, strong regulations were imposed on the marketing of beer, wine, and hard liquor. Federal regulators had to clear every ad for alcoholic beverages before it could run. Regulations and industry codes prohibited alcohol from being associated with women, patriotism, health, or any sort of glamorous activity. Neither wine nor liquor could be advertised on radio or television.

Over the past few decades these restraints have gradually been weakening. Today several of the largest beer manufacturers and importers—including Anheuser-Busch, Heublein, Schlitz, Coors, and Van Munching—are among the top advertisers on radio and television. Wine, too, is now advertised through these media. And no law explicitly bans the advertising of hard liquor on the air. "Given the permissive environment that has developed on so many other matters," says Stanley Cohen, Washington bureau chief of *Advertising Age*, "I assume it is only a matter of time before liquor will be on television, too."

The marketing of alcoholic beverages today is virtually indistinguishable from that of other products. Ads for alcoholic beverages are well researched, slickly produced, and backed by well-organized promotions at the retail level. Though the number of major brewers is dwindling, brands of beer are proliferating, many with their own advertising themes. "Alcoholic beverages have achieved respectability and are marketed by the same people and through the same channels as soap, Chevys, and cigarettes," says Cohen.

A good example of the new emphasis on marketing was the Coca-Cola Company's effect on the wine market. When Coca-Cola bought the Taylor brand of wines in the late 1970s, it set out to promote the image of wine as a drink that is consumed regularly rather than just on special occasions. Within a few years the amount of advertising in the wine industry nearly doubled—largely because of Coca-Cola's aggressive marketing techniques.

The tactics used to advertise alcohol differ little from those used with other products. Advertisements may indirectly associate drinking with wealth, success, or social approval. They may portray drinking as a sexy, sophisticated act. "As might be expected," says Wallack, "advertising seeks to place the product in the best possible light and is little, if at all, concerned with its possible adverse consequences."

The effect of such advertising remains a point of controversy. Researchers have never been able to agree on whether alcohol advertising increases the amount people drink or simply influences what brand of alcohol they buy. For instance, Mark Keller of Rutgers University contends that "you do not have to advertise alcohol to people. Why is the industry here spending millions on advertising? Because there is competition over who is going to sell how much of what. But I do not know whether advertising really increases the volume of consumption."

The National Research Council panel on alcohol abuse has also decided that the jury is still out on the influence of alcohol advertising. "It is generally thought that the main effect of commercial advertising is to alert the public to new brands, in competition with older ones, and conversely to protect or expand the market shares of established brands," the panel concludes. "The available scientific evidence is too sparse to permit us any extended discussion of the effects of advertising policies. Nevertheless, important issues of principle are involved in such policies."

These "issues of principle" may in fact be the most important aspect of the controversy surrounding alcohol advertising. Because such advertising is invariably enmeshed in the much broader social context of drinking, it may be impossible to study the effects of that advertising in isolation. The issue then becomes one of politics and public policy as much as scientific research. "The fundamental issue that we need to address is whether the wide-scale promotion of alcoholic beverages is consistent with the goals of a society concerned with minimizing the social, economic, and personal hardships associated with current levels of alcohol-related problems," says Wallack.

Voluntary Restraint by Industry

Despite the lack of hard evidence linking exposure to drinking or alcohol advertising to increased consumption, many groups and individuals have sought to limit the extent of these influences. Within the television and advertising industries themselves, many people are concerned about alcohol-related problems and ways to prevent them. This concern has in turn led to some innovative steps toward self-regulation.

In the television industry one of the most prominent developments of recent years has been the work of the Alcohol and Drug Abuse Committee of the Caucus of Producers, Writers, and Directors, a 160-member consortium of people involved in the creation of television shows. As with many individuals, the caucus was spurred into action by tragedy: In 1982 Natalie Wood and William Holden died in alcohol-related accidents, and an automobile accident caused by a drunk driver seriously injured Mary Martin and Janet Gaynor and killed Martin's manager.

A few months after these accidents the caucus issued a white paper entitled "We've Done Some Thinking." The paper asked whether "any of us as members of the creative community in Hollywood unwittingly glorified the casual use of alcohol in one of our projects? . . . The answer, we fear, is yes." According to Larry Stewart, chairman of the caucus's Alcohol and Drug Abuse Committee, the paper circulated widely in Hollywood. "Our committee has attempted to bring an idea to the attention of the creative community, and we feel confident that that community will respond on its own in a positive way," says Stewart. "We think we are sensible and that our colleagues are going to react sensibly."

The paper drew heavily on the research of Warren Breed and James Defoe, who had worked with such shows as "The Jeffersons," "M.A.S.H.," "All in the Family," and "One Day at a Time" to limit the amount of drinking shown. This process involves working directly with the scripts to monitor the ways in which drinking is portrayed. The white paper also included a number of suggestions for writers, producers, and directors, such as not glamorizing alcohol, substituting other beverages for alcohol when possible, demonstrating that people do not have to drink to be normal, portraying critical reactions to heavy drinking, dealing with the full range of consequences of drinking, and showing that there are no miraculous cures for alcoholism.

"We are not telling 'Love Boat' that they should not have a bar," says Stewart. "We are not telling 'Cheers' or 'Archie Bunker' to close down their sets because they take place in bars. But if drinking is not germane to the story, why show it? It if is germane, portray it, but do so with the awareness that the people we create become role models."

Such voluntary efforts also have a place in the advertising industry. An example is the Code of Advertising Standards developed by the Wine Institute, a trade association of 460 California vintners. The code emphasizes promoting wine responsibly, educating consumers about wine's heritage and moderate use, and participating in projects to reduce the misuse of alcohol. Specific parts of the code prohibit the use of athletes or celebrities attractive to young people, bar any suggestion of intoxication or drinking and driving, and discourage any association of wine with rites of passage.

All of the Wine Institute's 460 members, representing 95 percent of the California wine industry, voluntarily subscribe to the code. Furthermore, the Wine Institute has asked the Bureau of Alcohol, Tobacco, and Firearms to extend these provisions by law to all alcohol advertising.

Educational and Training Programs

The power of the mass media, so evident in the field of advertising, can also be turned to other purposes. In particular, the mass media are one of the best ways to convey health-related information about alcohol and the possible consequences of drinking. Such educational campaigns are often mentioned as part of a comprehensive program to prevent alcohol problems. Their potential strengths and weaknesses are the subject of the rest of this chapter.

Educational campaigns draw on the moral authority of the government or a respected private organization to try to persuade people to drink safely or appropriately. Generally, such programs have prestige and legitimacy in our society. However, even after decades of experience with educational campaigns, their effectiveness remains open to question. With some recent and notable exceptions, there is little hard evidence to show that past educational campaigns using the mass media have had any significant effect. Some people seem to pay no attention to the messages about health that they get through the media. Those who do pay attention are also those most likely to have their preexisting beliefs confirmed. For these and other reasons, many social scientists have concluded that mass media educational campaigns are doomed to fail.

Dissenting social scientists argue that past campaigns have been poorly planned, executed, or evaluated. They also point out that mass media campaigns are most effective when combined with other, reinforcing measures. "Given the lack of both formative research and sufficient evaluation, it is no wonder that previous public education campaigns aimed at reducing the incidence of alcohol abuse have had such inconclusive results," writes John Hochheimer of Stanford University. "Proper use of the mass media for effective dissemination of messages is a multifaceted process that requires a great deal of planning,

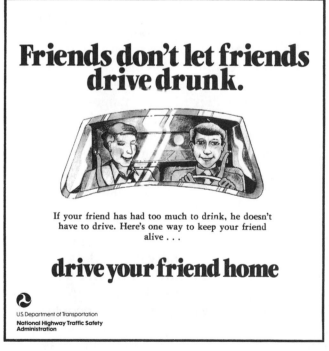

Suggestions for specific actions or behaviors tend to be more effective than general admonitions in mass media educational campaigns.

evaluation, and willingness to replan during the campaign if necessary."

At the same time, not all educational campaigns have been a failure. It is true that the most successful campaigns have focused on other health concerns, such as smoking or heart disease, rather than on drinking problems. Nevertheless, these efforts can give direction to an alcohol-related campaign. One such well-known program is the Three Community Study of the Stanford Heart Disease Prevention Project.

The Three Community Study set out to determine if state-of-the-art mass media programming could influence the factors associated with the risk of heart disease. The Department of Communication at Stanford University produced more than 50 television spots and more than 100 radio spots of 10 to 60 seconds' duration, plus more than three hours of television programming, many hours of radio programming, newspaper columns, advertisements, and direct mail.

These messages were designed to educate people about the risks of heart disease and to encourage them to reduce those risks through dietary changes, giving up cigarettes, a return to ideal weight, and programs of regular exercise. Wherever possible, the messages mentioned specific skills or techniques that people could use to achieve these changes.

In one of the two experimental towns in central California, the Three Community Study went beyond this mass media approach. Either at home or in formal classes, physicians and other health educators individually taught the people at highest risk of heart disease some specific skills that they could use to achieve a healthier lifestyle.

The results of the Three Community Study were striking. After two years the people in both experimental towns had average reductions in the overall estimated risk of heart disease of between 16 and 18 percent. In a control town the average risk *increased* 6.5 percent. Overall, the people in the experimental towns did not lose weight, but the people in the control town gained weight.

As expected, the town receiving both the mass media information and the intensive training had the largest initial overall reduction in risk. But by the end of two years, the town receiving only the mass media information had caught up with the town that also received the personalized training. Still, the training had a specific noticeable effect. In the control town and the town receiving only the mass media information, few people managed to quit smoking. But of the people who received individualized instruction, half of those who had been smokers quit.

There are many questions that would have to be answered before a program similar to the Three Community Study could be widely applied to alcohol problems. For instance, what is the best way to scale up a relatively small program to a national equivalent? In the Three Community Study, the organizers of the program were highly committed. In a national program of alcohol education, the organizations called upon to administer the program may initially be skeptical or indifferent. Nevertheless, the combination of mass media health information and personalized training is a promising one. Educational training programs on alcohol would be a valuable step forward, although at this stage their primary goal should be the collection of further research data.

Lessons for Future Educational Campaigns

The Three Community Study demonstrated several important rules that any similar program should follow. An important set of rules concerns the messages sent through the mass media. "A message should not try to be all things to all people," writes Hochheimer. "It should be targeted to a specific audience, which involves defining who that audience is, what those people are like, what it is we want to change, what the best strategy is to change it, and what is the most efficacious method of disseminating that information." This approach acknowledges "that the audience is an equal partner in the communication process," according to Hochheimer.

The source of the message is also important. The credibility, attractiveness, and forcefulness of the source all influence how much impact a message has. For instance, in some cases the government may not have much credibility as a source of health information, according to Hochheimer. The government's position should therefore be carefully studied in designing an educational campaign on alcohol-related problems. As another example, the use of older celebrities like Dick Van Dyke or Art Carney in educational campaigns about alcohol may have little relevance to younger people.

The message itself should be specific and to the point. Research shows that messages advocating a specific behavior are better than vague admonitions. Thus the message "If your friend is drunk at a party, take him home in his car and ask another friend to drive behind to pick you up" is better than "Friends don't let friends drive drunk," according to Hochheimer. Another example of a specific message is "Why not make every third drink a soft drink at the next party."

Messages that rely on fear—such as "Drunk drivers add color to our highways" or movies portraying the evils of alcohol or drug addiction—may backfire. If messages are too heavy-handed, people may ignore or avoid them to avoid feeling the emotions that such messages are supposed to engender. People may also see them as exaggerated and consequently dismiss less drastic messages as equally biased.

An educational campaign should also make use of a variety of different media. The obvious media are television, radio, and newspapers. But there are also billboards, direct mail, magazines, newsletters, films, subway and bus ads, and the insertion of materials into paychecks. These messages should be coordinated so that they reinforce each other and do not conflict. In addition, educational campaigns should draw on the professional knowledge and skills of people trained in the behavioral and communication sciences. Past programs that have relied exclusively on the expertise of commercial advertisers or the enthusiasm of local volunteer groups have generally not achieved their desired ends.

Finally, educational campaigns must do more than just supply people with information. They must suggest specific behaviors and teach specific skills that enable people to make changes that they want to make. If possible, this education can take the form of low-key training programs. There is even an institutional base that can support these programs—local hospitals and the rapidly expanding network of health maintenance organizations. These organizations can offer individualized training at a relatively low cost. They have the potential to make it relatively easy and, perhaps more important, relatively unembarrassing for people to learn ways to moderate their drinking.

With regard to the overall prospects for educational programs dealing with alcohol-related problems, the panel concluded, ". . . [T]here is potential in these areas, but it does not lie where we have commonly looked. It is not exclusively in the schools or in mass media advertising. It may be in information and training programs sponsored by universities and health maintenance organizations focusing on the health risks of some drinking practices and teaching techniques for modifying personal drinking habits."

The Conflict Between Education and Other Media Messages

As we saw in the first part of this chapter, educational programs using mass media may have a formidable barrier to overcome. They must rely at least in part on the media to convey their messages. Yet these same media also transmit many messages that implicitly or explicitly glamorize drinking. As a result, says Lawrence Wallack, alcohol educational campaigns "exist in a generally hostile environment rich with messages supporting and encouraging the use and misuse of alcohol. The major contributor to this antieducation environment is clearly alcoholic beverage advertising. The massive amount of misleading information being disseminated through alcoholic beverage advertising acts as a barrier to the success of community-based programs and larger public information efforts. Television programming is also a great, though inadvertent, contributor to this vast reservoir of misinformation."

One measure of the relative strengths of advertising and alcohol education is the resources devoted to each. In a recent year the National Institute on Alcohol Abuse and Alcoholism spent $11.4 million to provide information on alcohol to the public. Even if each of the states spent $1 million on similar efforts, the combined resources for public alcohol education—about $60 million—would equal only half of the advertising budgets of either the Anheuser-Busch or Miller brewing companies. Compared with the over $1 billion spent yearly on alcohol advertising, these public expenditures are almost insignificant.

There are several ways to narrow this gap. One is to increase funds for public alcohol education. Voluntary, self-initiated restraints, such as those advocated by the Caucus of Producers, Writers, and Directors and the Wine Institute, are a second approach. A third approach involves governmental legislation or regulation. This last approach, says Stanley Cohen, "requires a cohesive and realistic strategy. The odds are not attractive, but they are not impossible."

Wallack suggests two governmental policies that he sees as "a starting point for further discussion." The first is to withdraw the business tax deduction for advertising alcoholic beverages. An estimated $350 million of the $1 billion spent on alcohol advertising is now deducted from corporate taxes. Wallack's second suggestion is to levy a 10 percent tax on alcoholic beverage advertising to fund educational campaigns. This would be a way "to fund advertisements that show the other side of the alcoholic beverage story," he says.

Compared with the number of messages in the mass media that promote or glamorize drinking, an educational campaign can seem "a slim reed," in the words of Stanley Cohen. But an educational campaign does not have to act alone. Such campaigns can reinforce the many other forces in society that tend to moderate drinking. They can draw attention to laws that prohibit specific actions like drinking and driving. Or they can be a vehicle for some other way of preventing alcohol problems, such as individualized training. As part of a multifaceted program of prevention, educational campaigns can be both easier to get started and more effective once they are launched.

8

Reducing
Environmental
Risk

N O MATTER HOW EFFECTIVE an educational campaign, no
matter how the availability of alcohol is changed, some
people will still drink in dangerous, careless, or just un-
lucky ways. As a result, alcohol-related problems will always
occur. But there is another way to reduce the number or severity
of these problems. This third category of preventive instruments does not focus on how much or where people drink, as
do educational programs, increased taxation, and so on. Instead, these preventive actions ask how the physical and social
environment might be changed to protect people from the
harmful consequences of drinking.

Changing the environment rather than behavior has long
been seen as a way to protect people from their own actions,
and not only in the area of drinking. "When we have a dangerous traffic intersection we very seldom mount a campaign
to educate the public about the dangers of the intersection,"
says Robert Reynolds of San Diego County's Department of
Health Services. "Instead, we install a traffic light or in serious
instances we construct an overpass. In short, we alter the physical environment in lieu of attempting to modify individual
behavior through increased awareness of the problem."

Such steps to make the environment more forgiving benefit everyone, not just those who have been drinking. Drunkenness is only one of a number of impairments, including fatigue, absent-mindedness, illness, anger, or previous minor injuries, that can increase the danger in certain activities. If the world is made safer for people who have been drinking, it is made safer for everyone.

Changes in the Physical Environment

Accidents are a major cause of death in the United States. Approximately 100,000 people die each year as a result of accidents—about 1 in every 20 deaths. Many more people are left with serious injuries, some of which will impair them for the rest of their lives.

As noted in Chapter 3, roughly half of these 100,000 accidental deaths per year involve motor vehicles. But that leaves in excess of 50,000 deaths a year that are caused by other kinds of accidents—falls, fires, drownings, and so on. Limited studies have suggested that alcohol may be involved in as many—or more—of these deaths as in traffic accidents. This is a hard statistic to pin down, however, because blood alcohol measurements, which are routinely made after traffic accidents, are not as commonly made after other kinds of fatal accidents.

The most efficient physical devices now available for preventing accidental deaths are passive restraints in automobiles. If every automobile were equipped with airbags or automatic restraining belts, a substantial fraction of the people now killed in traffic accidents would be saved. Just how many people would be saved, and at what economic and social costs, have long been subjects of debate within government and the automobile industry.

Other environmental modifications could also have a significant effect on safety. An example is that of fires in homes caused by cigarettes and other smoking materials. According to James Mosher and Joseph Mottl of the University of California at Berkeley, residential fires caused by smoking "are surprisingly common in the United States." In 1978, according to the U.S. Fire Administration, some 70,000 smoking-related

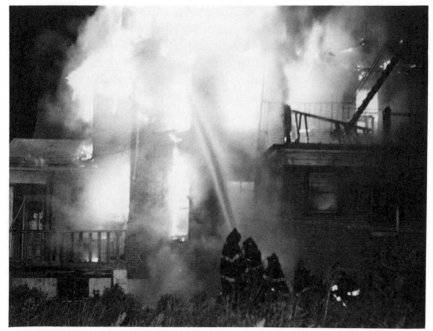

U.S. Fire Administration

Fires and other accidents kill as many people as do traffic accidents, and similar proportions of these deaths may be related to alcohol abuse.

fires caused 1,800 deaths, 4,000 injuries, and $180 million in economic losses. The U.S. per capita rate of fire deaths is one of the highest in the world. Moreover, note Mosher and Mottl, alcohol is involved in many of these deaths. In one study in Maryland, 67 percent of the people aged 30-59 killed in residential fires were legally drunk.

There are many ways to reduce the risk of residential fires in the United States. According to Mosher and Mottl, manufacturers of home furnishings and cigarettes do not use a variety of fireproofing techniques that are available. For instance, for several years the Consumer Product Safety Commission sought to institute regulations requiring that cigarettes be manufactured to go out if not smoked within a few minutes. These proposals were backed by most of the major fire prevention lobbying groups. But the cigarette industry exerted enough pressure to keep them from becoming law.

The debates over passive restraints in automobiles and self-extinguishing cigarettes are two examples of how public policy affecting safety is established in the United States. The process involves a delicate balancing of concern for the public, pressures from private industry, and general ideas about the role of government in society. It is a difficult, inevitably political process. Yet in the area of alcohol-related problems it determines the realm in which preventive initiatives will be able to take effect.

The Government's Role in Safety

Since the federal government passed the Pure Food and Drug Act in 1906, its involvement in various aspects of safety has continually increased. Today a variety of federal, state, and local governmental agencies are charged with safeguarding the public health. At the federal level these include the Occupational Safety and Health Administration, the Consumer Product Safety Commission, the Food and Drug Administration, the Environmental Protection Agency, the National Highway Traffic Safety Administration, the Nuclear Regulatory Commission, and the National Transportation Safety Board. Many other agencies within the federal government have also been given heightened responsibilities for safety.

This increased involvement with safety has had a measurable impact on mortality rates. "The federal concern for safety has made our society much safer than it was at the turn of the century in at least some regards," write Mosher and Mottl. "Working conditions in many industries have become less hazardous; dangerous pesticides and canning chemicals have been banned; the number of fatal accidents (including automobile deaths) has been reduced by nearly one-half proportionate to the population."

But this expansion of governmental oversight has not come without controversy. "While reducing potential risks of harm may be a proper goal for government, providing overprotection has its own social costs," write Mosher and Mottl. "Individual freedoms may be jeopardized; creativity, both of individuals and business, may be stifled; the viability of a small business may be eroded by the prohibitive costs of safety requirements.

Defining when and how to intervene to promote safety, then, is an important topic of current federal practice."

Consider the case of passive restraints in automobiles. The government has a number of options to try to encourage their use. It can educate consumers to buy or demand them. It can sponsor research to improve them. It can tax automobiles that do not have them. It can require that manufacturers offer them as options. It can require them outright. Or, if the government sees the costs of action as too high, it can do nothing.

Not all governmental initiatives involve as much controversy as do passive restraints in automobiles. In fact, Mosher and Mottl believe that many federal agencies are overlooking fairly straightforward ways to significantly reduce alcohol-related problems. In the field of transportation, for instance, several agencies—including the Department of Transportation, the Federal Aviation Administration, and the Coast Guard—recognize the role that alcohol plays in accidents yet have not moved forcefully to deal with the problem. "There appears to be a heavy emphasis on safety and a general recognition of alcohol involvement in transportation accidents among most of the federal agencies we studied," write Mosher and Mottl. "It is therefore surprising that there has been so little effort to evaluate the scope of the problem or to plan and implement programs to contend with it."

To some extent, these agencies are hamstrung by their own limited view of what can be done about alcohol problems. In general, safety-related federal agencies see alcoholism as the major problem to be addressed. When solutions are pursued, they almost invariably involve treatment and rehabilitation programs directed at alcoholics. Such treatment has little or no chance of affecting the many accidents that happen to people who are not alcoholics. Moreover, even when governmental agencies do become aware of preventive options, they may fail to act out of a belief that such initiatives are not included in their mandate.

One way to overcome these institutional barriers is through an oversight, coordinating, or watchdog body. Such an authority could encourage the relevant agencies or groups to take action where alcohol-related accidents are a problem. One example of such a body is the National Transportation Safety Board, which has a specific jurisdiction in the activities of a number of federal agencies. The National Institute on Alcohol Abuse and Alcoholism could be the logical site of a similar watchdog body focused on alcohol.

One of the first responsibilities of such a body should be to bring the same attention given to reporting blood alcohol content after traffic deaths to nontraffic deaths. This information would be a valuable guide in designing safer products and surroundings, not only for drinkers but for nondrinkers as well. Such an agency could also explore alternative policies to deal with alcohol-related problems, thus clarifying some of the trade-offs involved.

Public Drunkenness

Another important place where drinking and environmental factors intersect is in the laws and attitudes surrounding public drunkenness. There are two general justifications for such laws. The first is that they keep people who are drunk in public from harming or offending others. The second is that they keep these people from being the victims of crime, exposure, or illness.

These laws constitute one of the most significant involvements of the government in shaping drinking practices. According to the Federal Bureau of Investigation, over one million arrests are made each year for public intoxication. This offense and drunk driving are the two most common reasons for arrest in the United States.

In recent years a social movement has developed to decriminalize public drunkenness. This movement has argued that people drunk in public need social and medical services more than they need to be locked up in jail. To the extent that public violence and disorder related to alcohol use are a problem, laws against these offenses are more specific than blanket laws against drunkenness.

Persuaded by these arguments, about half of the cities and states in the United States have decriminalized public drunkenness. However, the actual way in which people drunk in public are handled has changed little. In many places, police are still the only public servants trained to handle such people. Even if intoxicants are now more often taken to detoxification units than to jail, they are still usually taken there by the police. Moreover, the police can hold people they pick up in protective custody before releasing them or transferring them to a treatment facility. Finally, the treatment facilities that were to provide the social and medical services still for the most part do not exist.

There are virtually no data on how the decriminalization of public drunkenness has affected public violence. In fact, the only clear effect of these changes has been the often repeated assertion that drunken people are more visible on city streets. Decriminalization does not seem to have made much difference to the health and welfare of chronic violators, though this may reflect the lack of services for them. It is possible that public drunkenness has increased, and that violence, vandalism, and disorder are associated with this increase. But the lack of studies in this area makes it almost impossible to suggest directions for reform.

The other side of the public drunkenness laws concerns the victimization of such people. Someone who is drunk in public is an easy mark for a criminal. As long as there has been drinking there have been jackrollers—people who mug and steal from drunken victims. Furthermore, American cities make it easier for jackrollers by concentrating their victims in certain districts.

There has been little discussion among the general public about such victimization. This is partly due to the issues of morality and culpability associated with intoxication. Drunkenness somehow seems to implicate the victim in the crime, to suggest that the victims deserve what they get. No one has yet studied the possible ways to shield people drunk in public from crime. It has not even been included in general accountings of the costs of alcohol abuse.

Some of the local, environmental approaches to public drunkenness that have been taken in the past may be a good starting point for such study. One problem is that urban renewal has demolished the traditional institutions of skid row, obliterating the old havens for impoverished drinkers. For several years

San Francisco used federal Model Cities money to run a "wet hotel," similar to the old municipal lodging houses. There the poor, like the rich, had a residential hotel in which they could drink. An improvement on this idea would be to offer the possibility of treatment on a voluntary basis through the facility. Those who continued to drink in the hotel could do so, but they could have access to care if they so desired.

Reducing Hostility Toward Drinking

Most adult Americans have been drunk or have been around someone who has been drunk. These experiences have probably helped to make many people hesitant to criticize or intervene in the drunken behavior of others. Given the potential of excessive drinking to cause harm, most people probably underreact to intoxication.

But the opposite situation can occur. People can use drinking as an excuse to deny another person's civil liberties or human rights. Hostility toward alcohol can reduce a drinker's normal opportunities for work or leisure. In some cases, a reduction in this hostility would be a step forward.

The most prominent area in which reducing hostility toward drinking could have a beneficial effect is that of recovery from alcoholism. Recovered alcoholics need tolerance and understanding as they try to reenter society. Even if they are currently abstemious, recovered alcoholics often face discrimination when looking for work and quickly learn to conceal their drinking histories. At the same time, this concern about stigmatization keeps some alcoholics from seeking treatment in the first place.

This prejudice against recovered alcoholics also has an institutional component. Until recently, the majority of health insurance plans did not cover treatment for alcoholism. Now this has begun to change. Laws in some states require that Blue Cross/Blue Shield cover alcoholism treatment. Other legislation forbids discrimination against alcoholics in housing and employment and regulates the confidentiality of medical records.

Another possible problem concerns attitudes about drinking in different parts of the country. The South, the Great Plains, and the mountain areas of the United States are much drier than the Northeast and West Coast regions. A nationwide governmental program to raise the level of concern about drinking may be out of place in these drier parts of the country. Similarly, someone who drinks in these parts of the country may feel unnecessarily condemned for doing so, although it is not known if this is a serious problem.

In general, there are potential risks in raising people's level of concern about their own and others' drinking. As more and more drinking behaviors are defined as unacceptable, the rate of those practices may decline. But the people who continue to drink in those ways will have a greater chance of being labeled as deviants and feeling at odds with the larger society. For some problems caused by drinking, it may be wiser to continue to deal with symptoms as they occasionally occur than to tackle an underlying cause.

9

Summary and Outlook

The easy problems in public health have mainly been solved. Alcohol-related problems are far more complicated and their solutions more fraught with trouble than when our predecessors tried to clean up the water supply, wipe out cholera and dysentery, and immunize people against smallpox. I do not mean to suggest that conquering smallpox and purifying the water supply were really easy. . . . But we see in alcohol-related problems a spectrum of considerations broader than any involved in the great achievements of public health in the past.

> William Mayer, former head of
> the Alcohol, Drug Abuse, and
> Mental Health Administration

*A*S *WILLIAM MAYER OBSERVES,* reducing the number of alcohol-related problems in America is a substantial challenge. In part, this is because of the prominent and deep-rooted role of drinking in American society (Chapter 1). Prohibition demonstrated that it is impossible to eliminate drinking in the United States. So, too, is it impossible to eliminate all of the problems caused by drinking—the accidents, the illnesses, the social and psychological impairments. But one of the major themes running through this book has been that these problems are not unassailable. Their extent can be made smaller or larger by taking or failing to take appropriate actions.

The links between drinking and the various consequences of drinking—both beneficial and detrimental—are exceedingly complex. Some of them depend on how much people drink, how their bodies react to alcohol, how often they drink, how much they drink altogether, where they drink, when they drink, what they do while and after they drink, and how risky the environment is in which they drink. This tangled web of cause and effect makes it difficult to design policies that reduce alcohol problems while not overly curtailing the positive consequences of drinking. But it can also be seen as an opportunity: Each separate link between drinking and its adverse consequences offers a different approach to dealing with alcohol-related problems.

An examination of which kinds of drinkers are susceptible to problems associated with alcohol reveals an unexpected finding (Chapter 2). Very heavy drinkers, including people generally considered alcoholics, do not suffer all of the problems caused by drinking. In fact, they do not even suffer most of them. Certainly, an alcoholic or heavy drinker has a greater chance of getting into trouble from drinking than does a more moderate drinker. But even a moderate drinker can be in an accident, become ill, or have difficulties with family or job that relate to drinking. Furthermore, there are many more moderate drinkers than heavy drinkers and many more heavy drinkers than alcoholics.

As a result, at least half of the alcohol-related problems that occur in the United States cannot be reached by treatment programs for alcoholics and other very heavy drinkers. It would be impossible to extend such programs to all drinkers. It would be too expensive, for one thing, and most light and moderate drinkers would justifiably feel that they don't need individualized treatment.

There is a different way to influence this sizable fraction of America's alcohol-related problems. It is through initiatives that seek to *prevent* such problems before they occur or become inevitable. Such initiatives differ in several fundamental ways from treatment programs for alcoholics. They are impersonal actions that apply uniformly to large groups of people, thus reaching many people for whom treatment would be inappropriate. To be effective, they should be light and unburdensome rather than powerful and controlling.

The most serious problem that preventive policies must face is drunk driving (Chapter 3). About half of the 44,000 people killed in 1984 in traffic accidents had alcohol in their blood. Not all of these traffic fatalities were caused solely by the intoxication of a driver. But researchers estimate that somewhere around a quarter of these lives could have been saved if no one ever drove after drinking. Similar estimates are that 150,000 to 300,000 disabling injuries and over $1 billion in property damage could be prevented annually by keeping people who have been drinking off the road.

Many of the preventive measures discussed in this book can help reduce drunk driving. But drunk drivers kill and injure enough innocent third parties to also require the intervention of the law. Research shows that raising the risk of arrest is a much more effective threat to potential drunk drivers than is imposing harsher penalties. An increased risk of arrest is especially important at night, when most of the traffic accidents caused by alcohol occur.

The other preventive measures considered in this book can be divided into three broad categories. In the first are those that affect the supply of alcohol and the places in which it is drunk. For the past 30 years, the price of alcohol and the restrictions on its availability have gradually been declining (Chapter 4). Because taxes on alcohol have not kept up with inflation, alcohol has become cheaper in real terms. Simultaneously, more outlets selling alcohol have opened, these outlets have kept longer hours, and reduced drinking ages have made alcohol available to more people. During this same period, per capita alcohol consumption has gone up in the United States, increasing by over 30 percent since 1950.

Research findings generally link increased consumption with lower real prices or increased availability. The evidence is now strong enough to urge caution upon legislators and Alcohol Beverage Control boards. For instance, studies have indicated that when taxes on alcohol go up, per capita consumption, cirrhosis death rates, and traffic fatalities all tend to go down. In making moves that will affect the price or availability of alcohol, decision makers should realize that their actions also influence the health and welfare of people who drink alcohol.

Another way to alter the supply of alcohol is by having commercial servers or social hosts see to it that their customers or guests do not drink too much or do not get in trouble if they do (Chapter 5). Server intervention is encouraged by dramshop laws in over half of the states. These laws make servers liable for damages if they serve an underage or "obviously intoxicated" person who later causes an accident. However, current dramshop laws have proven relatively ineffective. The term "obviously intoxicated" offers little guidance to servers or to members of a jury, and many servers have chosen simply to insure against dramshop liability rather than to take active measures to avoid it. Concerned groups and individuals have suggested that one way to make these laws more effective would be to rewrite them to recognize servers' overall degree of effort, including their willingness to intervene in the drinking of patrons and their efforts to see that patrons have a way to get home safely.

The second category of preventive measures focuses on the drinking practices of people once they have access to alcohol. Education, especially of school-age children, has long been seen as one way for society to shape these drinking practices in beneficial ways (Chapter 6). However, alcohol education in the schools has never been shown to have much effect. One problem may be that this education sets its sights too high. Young people have plenty of problems with alcohol while in school, including violence, peer pressure, accidents, and reduced classroom performance. Lessons that focused on these problems, perhaps by teaching ways to avoid them, could be more useful than lessons that seek to make people responsible drinkers for the rest of their lives.

There are many other forces in society that tend to moderate or increase drinking problems, including friends, family, and the mass media. Among the messages that may influence drinking are alcohol advertising and the frequent depiction of drinking on television (Chapter 7). However, as with violence on television, it is exceedingly difficult to conduct definitive research on the relationship between media depictions and real-life behavior.

The mass media can also be used to try to teach people that it is acceptable not to drink or that there are ways to drink more safely. Research shows, however, that isolated mass media campaigns have had little or no success in the past. A new approach that combines mass communication principles with individualized training for people who want to change has shown promise. But it is still uncertain if such efforts could be adapted to address alcohol-related problems on a large scale.

The third category of preventive measures considers ways to make drinking safer even if people don't change their drinking practices. This entails making changes in the physical or social environment to reduce the risk for people who drink and for those around them (Chapter 8). Because traffic fatalities account for about half of all the people killed in accidents, passive restraints in automobiles, including air bags and automatic seat belts, are the technological devices with the greatest potential to reduce alcohol-related accidental deaths. But as many people are killed in other kinds of accidents—falls, drownings, fires, etc.—as in traffic accidents, and alcohol may be involved in as many or more of these deaths. A more thorough accounting of alcohol's role in all accidental deaths and injuries would make it easier to design products, surroundings, tools, and vehicles that are safer for everyone, not just for people who have been drinking.

The quality of the evidence demonstrating the effectiveness of these various preventive measures differs. For changes in the price of alcohol and certain alterations in the physical environment, the evidence is fairly persuasive. For educational campaigns and changes in availability, the evidence is fragmentary or nonexistent.

It should be remembered, however, that each preventive initiative builds on the strength of all others. Another major theme of this book has been that prevention is a comprehensive concept, linking dozens of creative, well-balanced measures by the simple idea that they be broadly applied, impersonal, and properly directed. As Lawrence Wallack of the University of California at Berkeley says, "Too much comes out in the form, 'It is this or that' and not enough in the form, 'It is all of these things, and each has to be developed and constructed in relation to the development and construction of the others.' A single program in and of itself may not make a detectable difference, but in relation to other strategies, both individual and aggregate, every individual effort may in fact serve a very important function."

The Need for Community Support

The past few years have seen a tremendous outpouring of enthusiasm and support for prevention as a way to deal with alcohol-related problems. Many of the most innovative, vital, and effective measures that have been taken have at least one thing in common: they have been created and sustained at the community level:

• In San Francisco, where a petition from an oil company to permit alcoholic beverage sales at drive-through gas station minimarts became a rallying point around which individuals and groups gathered to confront alcohol problems—and eventually forced the withdrawal of the petition.

• In the south Bronx, where a community planning board has been working with state agencies to prevent the reestablishment of a high density of liquor stores in rebuilt areas.

• In Illinois, where community groups can draw upon two prevention resource centers for information, materials, and personnel to set up their own prevention programs.

• In the many corporations and other private companies that have found preventive programs to be cheaper than their share of the health care costs generated by alcohol abuse.

• In the over 100 chapters nationwide of Mothers Against Drunk Driving (MADD), in which people write letters, meet with local politicians, speak before community organizations, and otherwise work to achieve MADD's goals.

Movements like this, which largely concentrate on state and local initiatives, are well suited to today's political climate. Since the 1980 elections, many federal programs have been placed in block grants to the states. This has moved a great deal of the detailed decision making out of federal agencies and into the states. Interest has therefore intensified in prevention policies that can be implemented at the state and local levels.

The community is a particularly important focus of preventive efforts. By nature, prevention programs are either based in a community or must have support there to survive. This requires that the people of a community acknowledge that alcohol problems belong to everyone in the community, not just to the people directly afflicted. As Margaret Hastings of the Illinois Commission on Mental Health and Developmental Disabilities says, "Budgets for prevention programs are protected most effectively when there is community ownership of the idea—not just the schools or a parent group, but a consortium of community institutions. Then the chances that the prevention program will last are great."

Similarly, preventive initiatives that arise spontaneously within a community are the ones with the greatest chance of success. "Ultimately, action initiated within the community is the action most likely to seize the community agenda and provide the opportunity for successful community cooperation to reduce alcohol problems," says Robert Reynolds of San Diego County's Department of Health Services. "All too seldom are those interested in prevention policies able to capture the public's attention; we in the alcohol field must learn to respond with sensitivity, support, and creativity to the opportunities provided by others."

An important component of preventive measures instituted at the community level should be the sharing of information among groups and individuals pursuing similar aims. A wide variety of experiments are going on throughout the country in all three categories of prevention. As much as possible should be learned from these experiments. The National Institute on Alcohol Abuse and Alcoholism could take the lead in disseminating the results of these experiments and other information about prevention. Such a service could let people know what is possible and how to achieve it. According to Michael Fox of the Ohio General Assembly, "A resource that pulls together the social costs in the criminal justice system, the health care system, the drunk driving fatalities, the teenage population problems—that catalogs these costs and offers a menu from

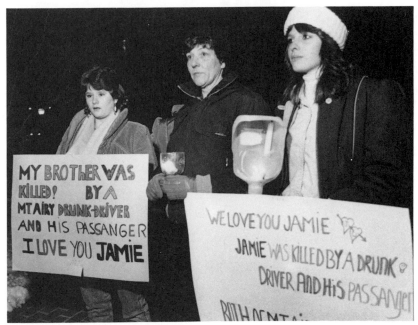

J. Henson, Capital Photo

A candlelight vigil organized by Mothers Against Drunk Driving (MADD). MADD and other groups like it are working to channel today's widespread concern about alcohol problems into specific legal and social actions.

which we can choose programs that have proven to be successful in a cost-effective way—would be extremely useful to policymakers, in the legislatures and state bureaucracies, and in county governments."

As more and more people learn about what prevention can do, its successes are likely to multiply. As Reynolds says, "Success tends to have a catalytic effect." When communities learn that they can deal with alcohol problems at a public beach or park, at a sports stadium, or at a neighborhood corner, they are more willing to take on additional or larger problems. People in the field of prevention have seen this happening, and they are working to encourage it.

It is an exciting time for the idea of prevention. Great energy and enthusiasm exist among many different groups and at many different levels. By putting these energies to use, a long-standing and serious problem in the United States could be significantly reduced. "Alcohol problems are now a topic of community discussion at the local, state, and national level," says Reynolds. ". . . This new social movement may well lead to major redefinitions of the role of alcohol in our society in the years ahead."

Guide to Information Sources

BOOKS

Alcohol and Health: Fifth Special Report to the U.S. Congress. U.S. Department of Health and Human Services. Washington, D.C.: U.S. Government Printing Office, 1983.

> A review of recent research on alcohol consumption and various categories of health problems. A final chapter, "Prevention: A Broad Perspective," discusses such topics as education, regulation, and the current activities of various organizations relevant to prevention.

Alcohol and Public Policy: Beyond the Shadow of Prohibition. Mark Moore and Dean Gerstein, eds. Washington, D.C.: National Academy Press, 1981.

> An examination by the Panel on Alternative Policies Affecting the Prevention of Alcohol Abuse and Alcoholism of the role prevention-oriented public policies can play in reducing alcohol-related problems in the United States.

Alcoholism, Alcohol Abuse, and Related Problems: Opportunities for Research. Division of Health Promotion and Disease Prevention, Institute of Medicine. Washington, D.C.: National Academy of Sciences, 1980.

> A wide-ranging assessment of the research needed to develop effective treatment and prevention programs for alcoholism and alcohol abuse.

Alcoholism and Related Problems: Issues for the American Public. Louis Jolyon West, ed. Englewood Cliffs, N. J.: Prentice-Hall, 1984.

> A collection of papers and consensus report from a 1984 session of the American Assembly of Columbia University examining the relation of

113

alcohol problems to issues in economics, law enforcement, prevention, treatment, and public policy.

The Alcohol Republic: An American Tradition. W. J. Rorabaugh. New York: Oxford University Press, 1979.

A historical analysis of drinking during the first 50 years of America's history, concluding with a look at the temperance movement of the 1830s, which dramatically reduced the high levels of consumption prevalent at that time.

Alcohol, Society, and the State. Vol. 1: *A Comparative Study of Alcohol Control.* Vol. 2: *The Social History of Control Policy in Seven Countries.* Toronto: Addiction Research Foundation, 1981.

An analysis conducted by the International Study of Alcohol Control Experiences in collaboration with the World Health Organization's Regional Office for Europe on the efforts of several industrialized countries to control alcohol sales and consumption since World War II.

Alcohol, Young Drivers, and Traffic Accidents. Alexander C. Wagenaar. Lexington, Mass.: D.C. Heath, 1983.

A review of how changes in the minimum drinking age, either up or down, have affected the involvement of young people in alcohol-related automobile crashes.

Annual Statistical Review 1983/84. Economics and Statistics Division, Distilled Spirits Council of the United States. Washington, D.C.: Distilled Spirits Council of the United States, 1984.

A compilation of statistics on the production, consumption, foreign trade, distribution, state and local control, and other aspects of the distilled spirits industry.

The Chemical People Book: A National School-Age Drug and Alcohol Abuse Campaign. Lloyd Kaiser, ed. Pittsburgh: QED Enterprises, 1983.

A guide and accompaniment to the campaign developed by public television station WQED in Pittsburgh to combat drug and alcohol abuse among school-age adolescents. The book details the steps and procedures by which the campaign formed thousands of local task forces.

The Culture of Public Problems: Drinking-Driving and the Symbolic Order. Joseph R. Gusfield. Chicago: University of Chicago Press, 1981.

A "research essay" on the cultural and social factors that encourage and discourage drunk driving in the United States.

Deliver Us From Evil: An Interpretation of American Prohibition. Norman H. Clark. New York: W.W. Norton, 1976.

A social history of America's most radical attempt to legislate drinking habits, considering both the effects of the prohibition movement on political history before 1916 and the legacies of Prohibition.

Deterring the Drinking Driver: Legal Policy and Social Control. H. Laurence Ross. Lexington, Mass.: D.C. Heath, 1984.

The revised and updated edition of a comprehensive overview of drinking and driving and especially of the factors that influence the effectiveness of drunk driving laws.

Driving the Drunk Off the Road. Sandy Golden. Washington, D.C.: Acropolis Books, 1983.

> An action-oriented guide for private citizens and government. The establishment of a Students Against Drunk Driving group is presented as a model, and individual chapters discuss how to use the media to help bring about drunk-driving reform, how to work with elected officials, and how to establish and contribute to state and local task groups.

Economics and Alcohol: Consumption and Control. Marcus Grant, Martin Plant, and Alan Williams, eds. New York: Gardner Press, 1983.

> A collection of papers exploring the nature and strength of the link between economic factors and alcohol use and abuse, demonstrating both the potential and limitations of economic analyses in alcohol-related areas.

Toward the Prevention of Alcohol Problems: Government, Business, and Community Action. Dean Gerstein, ed. Washington, D.C: National Academy Press, 1984.

> A summary of a 1983 conference held under the auspices of the Panel on Alternative Policies Affecting the Prevention of Alcohol Abuse and Alcoholism to discuss and expand upon the issues presented in *Alcohol and Public Policy: Beyond the Shadow of Prohibition.*

Will America Sober Up? Allan Luks. Boston: Beacon Press, 1983.

> An examination of current trends and developments in the area of prevention. Individual chapters discuss public policies geared toward prevention, dealcoholized beverages, and new research on alcoholism.

ORGANIZATIONS

Alcoholism Report, Inc., 1511 K Street, N.W., Suite 314, Washington, DC 20005.

> Publisher of *Alcoholism Report*, a semimonthly newsletter that covers legislative and policy developments at the national level affecting the alcohol and drug fields.

Alcohol Research Information Service, 1120 East Oakland Avenue, Lansing, MI 48906.

> A nonprofit organization whose purpose is to collect, correlate, and disseminate information on alcohol and alcoholic products; their manufacture, sale, and use for beverage, industrial, or other purposes; and their relation to the health and well-being of people in the United States.

Center for Science in the Public Interest, 1501 Sixteenth Street, N.W., Washington, DC 20036.

> Coordinator of the Project to Stop Marketing Alcohol on Radio and Television. Project SMART is a national petition campaign calling on Congress either to ban all alcohol advertising on television and radio or to require equal broadcast time for health and safety messages about drinking.

Council on Alcohol Policy, c/o The Trauma Foundation, Building 1, San Francisco General Hospital, San Francisco, CA 94110.

> One of nine councils of the National Association for Public Health Policy. The purpose of the council is to develop and implement sound public-health-oriented alcohol policy at state and federal levels.

Distilled Spirits Council of the United States, 1250 Eye Street, N.W., Suite 900, Washington, DC 20005.

> The national trade association of the domestic distilled spirits industry. DISCUS provides information, monitors the laws affecting the industry at all governmental levels, conducts public awareness and educational programs to encourage the responsible use of distilled spirits, and promotes sound business practices within the industry.

Mothers Against Drunk Driving, 669 Airport Freeway, Suite 310, Hurst, TX 76053.

> The national headquarters of MADD, which has over 300 chapters at state and local levels.

National Clearinghouse for Alcohol Information, P.O. Box 2345, Rockville, MD 20852.

> The information service of the National Institute for Alcohol Abuse and Alcoholism. The clearinghouse provides up-to-date information about a wide range of alcohol issues, including prevention, both upon request and through regular publications.

National Council on Alcoholism, 12 West Twenty-First Street, New York,NY 10010.

> A national voluntary health agency that focuses on the treatment and prevention of alcoholism and alcohol abuse through public education and advocacy. Nearly 200 local and state affiliates provide information about alcoholism, treatment opportunities, and prevention.

National Highway Traffic Safety Administration, Office of Alcohol Countermeasures, 400 Seventh Street, S.W., Washington, DC 20590.

> The division within the federal government that provides resources and technical assistance to state and local drunk driving programs and activities.

New York State Division of Alcoholism and Alcohol Abuse, 194 Washington Avenue, Albany, NY 12210.

> The agency within New York State that deals with alcoholism and alcohol abuse. The division has been particularly active in the areas of prevention, intervention, and education. Every state government contains a similar agency that directs alcohol programs at the state, county, or local levels and maintains liaisons with other organizations in the same field.

Prevention Research Center, 2532 Durant Avenue, Berkeley, CA 94704.

> One of nine national alcohol research institutes in the United States. The center conducts research on prevention issues, holds monthly seminars, and reports on current knowledge about prevention research to professional, academic, and community audiences.

San Diego County Department of Health Services—Alcohol Program, 3851 Rosecrans Street, San Diego, CA 92110.

A countywide alcohol program that has been particularly active in seeking community-based solutions to alcohol problems and in organizing and implementing prevention initiatives.

U.S. Brewers Association, 1750 K Street, N.W., Washington, DC 20006.

The national trade association of domestic brewers and suppliers to the industry. The association follows the laws affecting the brewing industry and provides information to its members and the public concerning the industry and its products.

Wine Institute, 165 Post Street, San Francisco, CA 94108.

The trade association of California vintners, representing over 500 wine makers and several thousand growers in the state. The Wine Institute promotes the proper use of wine as a table beverage to accompany food and participates in community demonstration projects designed to reduce alcohol problems and to educate the public about alcoholism.

Panel on Alternative Policies Affecting the Prevention of Alcohol Abuse and Alcoholism

MARK H. MOORE (*Chair*), John F. Kennedy School of Government, Harvard University

GAIL BURTON ALLEN, Department of Psychiatry, St. Luke's-Roosevelt Hospital Center, New York

DAN E. BEAUCHAMP, Department of Health Policy and Administration, School of Public Health, University of North Carolina

PHILIP COOK, Institute of Policy Sciences and Public Affairs and Department of Economics, Duke University

JOHN KAPLAN, School of Law, Stanford University

NATHAN MACCOBY, Institute for Communication Research, Stanford University

DAVID MUSTO, Child Study Center and Department of History, Yale University

ROBIN ROOM, School of Public Health, University of California, Berkeley, and Medical Research Institute of San Francisco

THOMAS C. SCHELLING, John F. Kennedy School of Government, Harvard University

WOLFGANG SCHMIDT, Social Sciences Department, Alcoholism and Drug Addiction Research Foundation, Toronto

NORMAN SCOTCH, School of Public Health, and Department of Sociomedical Sciences and Community Medicine, School of Medicine, Boston University

DONALD J. TREIMAN, Department of Sociology, University of California, Los Angeles

JACQUELINE P. WISEMAN, Department of Sociology, University of California, San Diego

Index

A

Accidents, 15, 96
  automobile, 15, 32–34, 72–73,
    87, 106, 108
  celebrity victims, 87
  residential fires, 96–97
Adolescent drinking, 26, 70–81
  minimum drinking ages, 25,
    40–41, 47, 48, 56, 72–74, 106
  parental responsibilities, 76–77
  reasons for, 70–72
  schools' role, 74–76, 78–81,
    107
  traffic accident statistics, 72–73
  See also Drinking
Advertising, 48, 65, 107
  beer and wine, 85, 88
  distilled liquor, 83, 85
  expenditures, 93–94
  industry restraint, 88
  strategies and effects, 84–86
  taxation of expenditures, 94
  See also Mass media; Television
    programming and advertis-
    ing
Age. *See* Drinking age
Air bags, 43, 96, 108
Alcohol Act of 1969 (Finland),
    57–58

Alcohol and Drug Abuse Com-
    mittee, 87
Alcohol availability and price, 25,
    26, 45–61
  consumption relationship, 46–
    47, 49–53, 106–107
  drunk driving relationship, 40–
    41
  government regulation, 47–49
  limits on availability, 56–59
  political considerations, 59–61
  price decline, 45–46
  tax increases, 53–56
Alcohol Beverage Control (ABC)
    boards, 49
Alcohol consumption. *See* Drink-
    ing
Alcohol, Drug Abuse, and Men-
    tal Health Administration, 8
Alcohol Safety Action Projects,
    36, 38
Alcoholic beverage industry, 18,
    59–60
Alcoholics, discrimination
    against, 102
Alcoholics Anonymous, 8
Alcoholism, 8–10, 74
Anti-Saloon League, 6–7
Attitude changes

public drunkenness, 101
toward drinking, 4–9, 102–103
toward drunk driving, 38–39
Automobile accidents, 15, 32–34,
72–73, 87, 106, 108
Automobile protective devices,
42–43, 96, 98, 99, 108
air bags, 43, 96, 108
seat belts, 43, 96, 108

B

Bartender training, 63–65, 79
See also Server intervention
Beer
advertisements, 85
ethyl alcohol content, 10
taxes on, 45, 53–54
Blood alcohol concentration
(BAC), 11, 15, 96, 100
legal intoxication, 11, 34
Blue Cross/Blue Shield, 102
British Road Safety Act, 35–36
Bureau of Alcohol, Tobacco, and
Firearms, 48, 88

C

California, 63–65, 68, 76, 88, 90,
102, 109
Cancer, 16
Cardiovascular diseases, 16
Caucus of Producers, Writers,
and Directors, 87, 94
Cigarettes. *See* Smoking
Cirrhosis, 14–15, 51–53, 55
Coast Guard, 99
Coca-Cola Co., 85
Code of Advertising Standards,
88
College programs, 78–81
Colonial period, 4–5, 9
Commercial servers. *See* Server
intervention
Consumer Product Safety Com-
mission, 97, 98

Consumption of alcohol. *See*
Drinking

D

Decriminalization of public
drunkenness, 100–102
Defense Department, 30, 48
Demonstration Alcohol Education Project, 78–81
Denmark, 51
de Tocqueville, Alexis, 5
Diabetes, 16
District of Columbia, 48, 65, 72
Dramshop laws, 41, 62–63, 67–
68, 107
Drinking
alcohol availability and price
effects on, 46–47, 49–53
changes in drinking practices,
3
consumption measurement,
10–13
distribution of alcohol-related
problems, 21–24
emotional effects of, 17–18
fatalities related to, 13–18, 87,
96–98
health care costs, 17
health, effects on, 14–15, 16,
17, 19, 51–53, 55
historical and contemporary
perspectives, 1, 4–9, 18–19
income-level relationship, 56
metabolism rates, 11
per capita consumption, 2, 13,
46, 50, 106
positive effects, 18–19
See also Adolescent drinking
Drinking age, 25, 40–41, 47, 48,
56, 72–74, 106
Drug abuse, 15, 75
Drunk driving, 32–44, 106
alcohol availability effect on,
40–41
alcohol price effect on, 40, 52

arrests effect on, 34–38, 106
automobile protective devices,
  42–43
educational campaigns, 41–42
fatality statistics, 15, 32–34,
  72–73, 87, 106, 108
penalties effect on, 38–40

E

Education programs, 25–26
  mass media campaigns, 41–42,
    88–94, 108
  school programs, 74–76, 78–
    81, 107
Eighteenth Amendment, 1, 6
Environmental changes, 26, 95–
  103, 108
  automobile protective devices,
    42–43, 96, 98, 99, 108
  government role, 98–100
  location and design of drink-
    ing establishments, 65–67
Environmental Protection
  Agency, 98
Ethyl alcohol, 10

F

Federal Aviation Administration,
  99
Fetal alcohol syndrome, 16
Finland, 57–58
Fires, residential, 96–97
Food and Drug Administration,
  98

G

Government regulation, 27, 30–
  31, 69
  of alcohol sales, 47–49
  Prohibition era, 1–3, 6–8
  safety requirements, 98–100
  See also Taxation of alcohol

H

Happy hours, 65
Health, 14–15, 16, 17, 19, 51–53,
  55
Health and Human Services,
  Department of, 30
Health Education Foundation, 65
Homicide, 15
Hours of sale, 47, 48, 56

I

Illinois, 109
Insurance policies, 67–68, 102
Internal Revenue Service, 30, 48
Intoxicated customers. *See* Server
  intervention
Iowa, 63
Ischemic heart disease, 19

L

Legal actions, 25
  arrests and penalties for drunk
    driving, 34–40, 106
  dramshop laws, 41, 62–63, 67–
    68, 107
  drinking age, 40–41, 47, 48,
    56, 72–74, 106
  public drunkenness, 100–102
  See also Alcohol availability and
    price
Liability. *See* Server intervention
Liability insurance, 67–68
Licensing systems, 48–49
Liquor, distilled
  advertisements, 83, 85
  ethyl alcohol content, 10
  taxes on, 45, 53–54
Liver disease (cirrhosis), 14–15,
  51–53, 55
Liver metabolism, 11

M

Maryland, 97
Mass media, 24, 26, 39, 82–94

and adolescent drinking, 71–72
advertising strategies and effects, 84–86
conflicting messages, 93–94
drinking images presented by, 82–84, 107
education programs, 41–42, 88–93, 108
industry restraints, 86–88
See also Advertising; Television programming and advertising
Massachusetts, 65
Massachusetts University, 78–81
Minimum drinking age. *See* Drinking age
Minnesota University, 65
Mothers Against Drunk Driving (MADD), 30, 64, 65, 73, 109

N

National Center for Alcohol Education, 75
National Clearinghouse for Alcohol Information, 75
National Highway Traffic Safety Administration, 64, 73–74, 98
National Institute on Alcohol Abuse and Alcoholism, 8, 69, 74–75, 93, 100, 110
National Park Service, 30
National Transportation Safety Board, 98, 100
New York, 60, 65, 109
Noncommercial servers, 62
Nuclear Regulatory Commission, 98

O

Occupational Safety and Health Administration, 98
Organic brain syndromes, 17
Overdose of alcohol, 15

P

Parental responsibilities, 76–77
Pregnancy, and excessive alcohol consumption, 16
Presidential Commission on Drunk Driving, 30
Presidential Task Force on Drunk Driving, 64
Prevention policies, 20–31, 104–112
current initiatives, 29–31, 109–112
focus of, 3–4, 20–24, 104–106
objections and barriers to, 27–29
program elements, 24–26, 106–109
Price of alcohol. *See* Alcohol availability and price
Prohibition period, 1–3, 6–8, 49, 51, 104
Public drunkenness, 25, 100–102
Pure Food and Drug Act of 1906, 98

R

Remove Intoxicated Drivers (RID), 30, 73
Residential fires, 96–97
Road Safety Act of 1967 (Britain), 35–36

S

S&A Restaurant Corporation, 68–69
Safety Action Program, 79
San Francisco, 102, 109
School programs, 74–76, 78–81, 107
Seat belts, 43, 96, 108
Server intervention, 25, 62–69
bartender training, 63–65, 79
dramshop laws, 41, 62–63, 67–68, 107

drunk driving relationship, 41
liability, 67–68
program strategies, 65–69
Shalom program, 76
Small Business Administration, 48
Smoking, 17
cigarette tax, 59
residential fires, 96–97
Social relationships, 18
Spirits. *See* Liquor, distilled
Stanford University, 90
Strokes, 16
Student Opportunity Program, 79
Students Against Drunk Driving (SADD), 30, 73
Suicide, 15

T

Taxation of alcohol
alcohol consumption relationship, 51–53, 106
as major source of government revenue, 47–48
political considerations, 59–61
static level of, 45, 50
tax increases, 53–56
taxation of advertising expenditures, 94
See also Government regulation
Teenage drinking. *See* Adolescent drinking
Television programming and advertising, 82–84, 86–88, 93, 107
See also Advertising; Mass media
Temperance societies and theories, 5–6
Three Community Study, 90–91
Transportation
automobile protective devices, 42–43, 96, 98, 99, 108
government role in safety, 99
traffic accident statistics, 15, 32–34, 72–73, 106, 108
Transportation Department, 36, 99
Treatment programs, 24
health insurance, 102
Twenty-first Amendment, 2, 8, 48

V

Volstead Act, 7

W

Wine
advertisements, 85, 88
ethyl alcohol content, 10
taxes on, 45, 53–54
Wine Institute, 88, 94
Wisconsin, 64, 67

Z

Zoning laws, 57

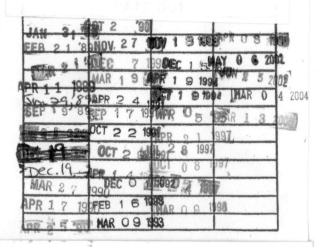